In a LITTLE KINGDOM

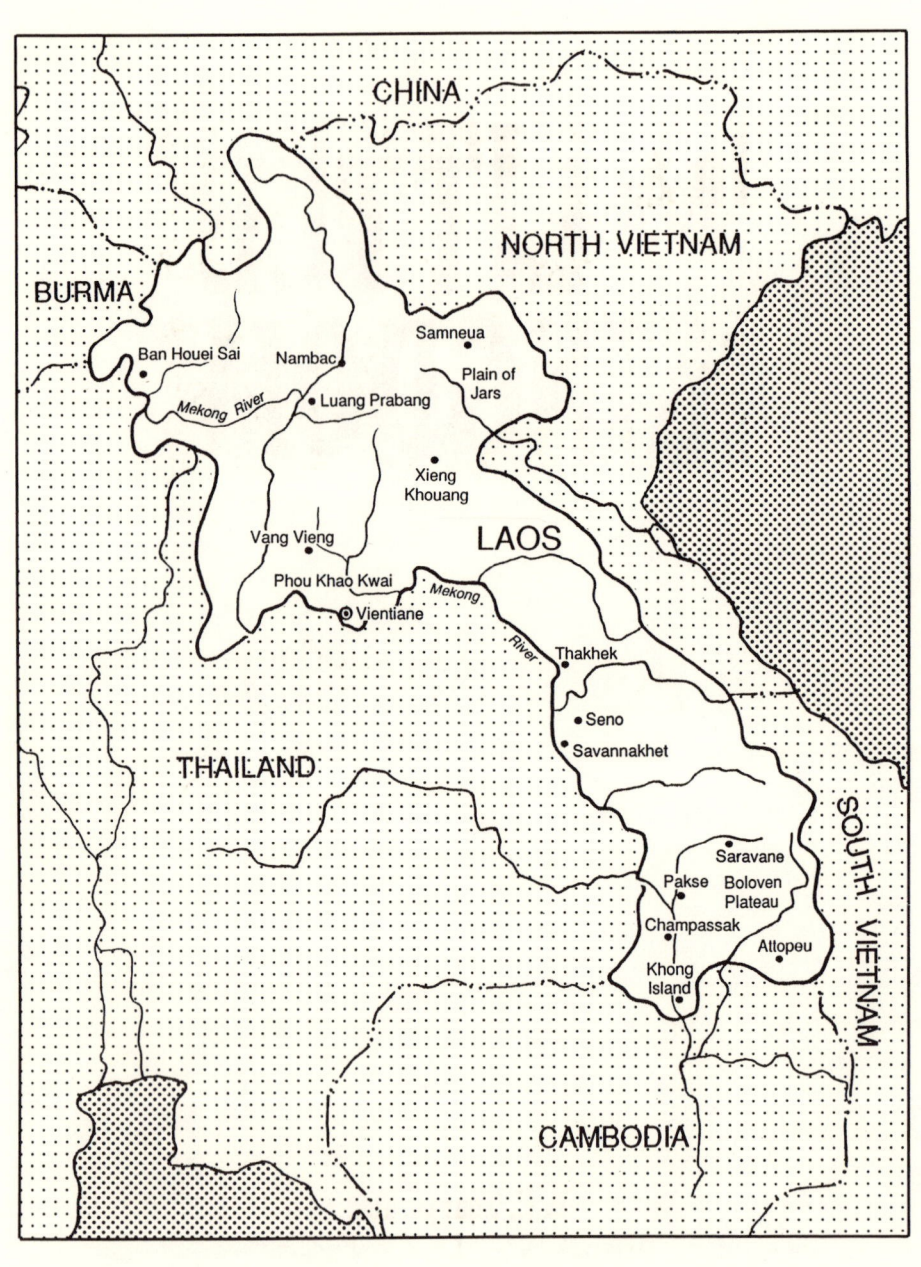

In a LITTLE KINGDOM

Perry Stieglitz

M.E. Sharpe, Inc.
Armonk, N.Y.   London, England

Library of Congress Cataloging-in-Publication Data

Stieglitz, Perry.
    In a little kingdom / by Perry Stieglitz.
      p. cm.
    ISBN 0-87332-617-2
    1. United States—Relations—Laos. 2. Laos—Relations—United States.
3. Stieglitz, Perry. 4. Americans—Laos—Biography. 5. Teachers—Laos—
Biography. I. Title
    E183.8.L28S75   1990
    303.48′2730594—dc20   90-8069
                                        CIP

For Moune

Contents

Preface

I first went there as a grantee, to teach for a year, but ever since I have been involved with Laos and it with me.

During its last decades, the Kingdom of Laos was inhabited by a gentle people with a few astonishingly able leaders. When the Vietnamese war monopolized American headlines, the little country became famous for the wrong reasons.

This book was conceived as an attempt to tell of the Laos I knew: its people, its culture, its history. I do not want the kingdom to disappear without some written record of why it was so special.

Many offered their efforts and enthusiasm to bring forth this work, and I am particularly thankful to Ruth Adams Paepcke, Richard Bartel, Joan Larson Kelly, and Gail Schlegel. Tribute must also be paid to three remarkable persons who in more recent years have each played a role in my life that has helped make this book possible: Ambassador Anne Cox Chambers, Chief Minister of Gibraltar Joseph Bossano, and the late Princess Chumbhot of Thailand. And then, of course, there are those numerous people mentioned in the book, to whom I shall always be grateful.

I

There Were Three Princes

1959–1961

I t is March 1959, and the setting is Hunter College High School, an academic institution reserved for the most intellectually gifted girls of New York City. One of the shining students was doing an *explication de texte* of a passage from Eliot's *Four Quartets*, and doing it very well, when a woman from the registrar's office entered the classroom with a message for me, the teacher. I employ the word *teacher* in this instance with some reluctance, for in this school we had to live with the realization that our students were apt to be far more gifted than we were, and our role tended to be less to teach than to encourage.

The message: a State Department official had telephoned from Washington to speak to me. The normal reaction would have been to dash off to the nearest phone. However, at Hunter High one did not dismiss a class lightly.

When the buzzer sounded I hurried down the hall, harboring the hope of getting back to French-speaking Europe, where I had done my graduate studies. Upon receiving tenure at Hunter, I had at once applied for a Fulbright grant to teach in France for a year. The application had been made in October. This must surely be the answer, and that it was coming by phone rather than mail indicated glad tidings.

But when I reached the man in Washington, he told me crisply and flatly that what I was being offered was a grant to teach English at the *lycée* of Vientiane in Laos.

"Laos?"

He enunciated as though for a dull pupil: "The Kingdom of Laos in Indochina."

"But what about France?" I demanded. "I applied for a teaching grant to France."

"You're not being offered France, you're being offered a position in Laos. We need a French-speaking teacher of English. Do you accept?"

I was a bachelor. I thought for perhaps twenty seconds and then accepted.

In the college library there were a few—not many—books and

magazine and newspaper articles pertaining to Laos. On a terrestrial globe, I found the little kingdom surrounded by Thailand, Burma, China, Vietnam, and Cambodia. It was inland, with no ready access to the sea. But the Mekong River, flowing down from China, formed a major part of the country's frontier with Thailand. The kingdom's cities were completely unknown to me—Vientiane, Savannakhet, Pakse, and Luang Prabang. Slowly spinning the sphere, I noticed that Laos was halfway around the circumference from New York—it could hardly have been farther away. In my escapist mood, the idea appealed.

❋ ❋ ❋

Here is a simplified, abbreviated version of what history books relate. The Kingdom of Lan Xang, or the Kingdom of a Million Elephants, existed until the end of the seventeenth century, when a period of warfare rent it into several smaller kingdoms, principally those of Luang Prabang and Champassak.

Two hundred years later, the French advanced into Southeast Asia and seized these various realms to create out of them the Kingdom of Laos. The conquerors then included Laos, along with Vietnam and Cambodia, in their great colony of French Indochina.

The Japanese occupied Indochina during World War II, and at a the end of the hostilities, for obvious reasons, hurriedly departed. The French hastened back to reclaim their colony, but the inevitable had happened: these countries had whiffed the air of independence and sought it for themselves. They were willing to go to war for their freedom.

However, as history warns, small kingdoms, poorly defended, fall prey to stronger nations.

◆ ◆ ◆

In the months that followed notification of my grant, if the little kingdom did not become exactly a household name, it did grow remarkably in the space allotted to it in the media. During August, while I was making final preparations for departure, my local newspaper, *The New York Times*, published more than seventy stories about Laos, some on the first page.

The reason for the kingdom's sudden fame was that although it had only recently achieved its independence, it was small and weak and had the misfortune to have the North Vietnamese as immediate neighbors. Vietnamese incursions had begun, and Vientiane was making appeals for assistance to the United States and other powers. Friends and family became concerned that I was heading for a war zone.

My flight across the Pacific was via Japan Air Lines and first class because in those days the State Department had all of its officers and grantees travel first class. Restless during the long night's flight, I stood for a while by the coffee bar and got into conversation with a fellow passenger, the readily recognizable Joseph Alsop. He asked me where I was going, and when I told him he unequivocally stated: "Young man, you won't be in Laos for more than a few months. Circumstances will not permit."

Alsop was wrong, but in defense of his powers of prognostication, let us note that within a week of his remark, the government of Laos did announce a state of emergency.

◆ ◆ ◆

The Royal Lao Airlines plane, a World War II veteran, traveled from Bangkok at sufficiently low height and speed to permit passengers a glimpse of villages and rice paddies interspersed through the otherwise lushly green landscape of Thailand. The passengers were both Asian and Western, and our comely stewardesses were elegant in their woven silk costumes. After some ninety minutes, the plane reached the broad and sinuous Mekong, and I had my first glimpse of Vientiane as it spread across the other side of the river. This was the first day of September 1959.

The airport, which turned out to be the nation's only major port, was neither exotic nor imposing. The simple wooden terminal appeared ramshackle. As the plane came to a halt, a swarm of people emerged from the structure's shade to surround the craft. Each passenger seemed to have his own welcoming contingent.

When I descended the ladder, a tall, heavy, blond American advanced. "Perry Stieglitz?" It was a declaration in the form of a question. He was in his early thirties with a most genial manner and a cherubic smile. His name was Charlie Searles, and he was the cultural attaché of the American embassy. Charlie had his driver take my baggage directly from the plane to his waiting jeep. The three of us mounted and drove off, my bags never having gone through customs.

The avenue was wide and thickly lined with heavily leafed rain trees. It was also crowded with cars, pedicabs, and bicycles. As we approached the main part of the city, where two-storied houses served as centers of commerce, there was a wide assortment of pedestrians.

What gave the city its unmistakable distinction were the temples, or *wats*, which were always set back from the road on green lawns. Tall cream-colored buildings with often lavishly carved wooden doorways, they were notable for their superb tiered roofs, sharply slanting down and then, near the edge, curving delicately up, their corners melting into thin sculpted wooden naga heads floating skyward. On the lawns of the *wats*, the monks, or *bonzes*, strolled serenely in their saffron robes.

The street along which we rode paralleled the river. But at the king's Vientiane palace, we turned away from the river and proceeded up the city's widest and most important thoroughfare, the Avenue Lan Xang. We passed *wats*, shops, houses, and the vast morning market. Beyond that was the *lycée* and the large traffic circle about which the National Assembly and other government buildings were situated.

I was finding the city enchanting until we turned to the right on a small unattractive road and stopped in front of a dreary, two-story, barracks-like building. This, Charlie informed me, was where my apartment was.

My lodgings, on the second floor, consisted of a room with shabby chairs and a desk separated by a partition of sorts from a large bed with torn mosquito netting draped around it. The facilities were out on the narrow back porch. At least, there was electricity—albeit eccentric—and running water and a flush toilet. There were no cooking possibilities, but I was advised that only fifteen minutes away by foot was the USAID compound, which had an institutional-type restaurant and where, Charlie told me, I had been given permission to eat. And this was in the rainy season.

If I had been in the Peace Corps, I might have been prepared for this or worse, but I felt that as a Fulbright teacher I should have been offered something better. And a search for other lodgings proved fruitless.

Later, when I had changed the furniture and the mosquito netting and bought lamps with shades that bathed the room in a dim, mysterious glow, a few visitors went so far as to suggest that it was an attractive flat.

For transportation, I bought a bicycle. I am told that riding a bike is good exercise, but cycling among the pedicabs and thousands of bikes in Vientiane is not good for the nerves.

◆ ◆ ◆

I wanted to get to know the Lao, but the people I initially met in Vientiane were Americans attached to the mission or the French who made up the world of the *lycée*.

The *Lycée de Vientiane* was remarkably handsome. It was situated on a large green campus, and its classrooms were contained in long buildings spread out about the campus. Each room opened onto the paths and lawns. Only the administration building, which housed the offices, the auditorium, and the faculty room, faced the Avenue Lan Xang. One could stroll on the campus and feel quite removed from nearby traffic.

The fall semester began, and I learned that I was about to become the first American ever tolerated on its faculty. The directors and other teachers were all French, with the exception of three Lao instructors. The studies prepared the pupils for the same *baccalauréat* exams given at the *lycées* in Paris. To teach English, I had to follow the French texts.

In Washington I had been told that I would be assigned to the advanced English courses. In Vientiane the French director, suspicious of the first American teacher foisted upon him, assigned me to six beginners' classes, with approximately thirty youngsters in each class. Fortunately, these children were for the most part calmer and quieter than my Hunter girls and often displayed a pleasant sense of humor.

Sometimes, while teaching a lesson, I would think how splendid it was that these boys and girls were being given a classical French education. Then I would decide how ridiculous: the textbook examples of life in French cities and villages were so removed from the experiences of these young Lao. Why should this be forced upon them?

Some of the faculty had been in Vientiane for many years. They spent nine months at the school and the remainder of the year on vacation in France, their traveling done at the French government's expense. It was a special way of life that appealed to them. Frequently, however, their remarks indicated that they still considered Laos a colony.

One French tradition scrupulously observed was that each morning upon entering the faculty room one had to shake hands with everyone in the room, even though they numbered twenty-five or more.

◆ ◆ ◆

Michelle was a senior political officer at the American embassy. A brilliant woman, fortyish, severe looking with a high forehead and a hearty laugh, she charmed the foreign diplomats but could scarcely abide most of her fellow Americans. Even though she was exceptional in performing her duties, the efficiency reports written about her contained devastatingly negative notes, a reflection on how people dislike being disliked.

Michelle happened to be of French background and a Francophile. She was predisposed to favor me, for I spoke French, I had studied in France, and I was an American teaching at the French *lycée*.

She befriended me, and I was delighted to spend time in her company. There was nothing simple about the political situation in Laos, and no one seemed better able to understand its intricacies than she was. She knew personally many of the Lao leaders, and since all of them spoke French, she spoke their language. She was given to making predictions with uncanny accuracy about how they were going to react as events occurred.

Michelle treated me in grand fashion. She did not slight me because I was merely a grantee. She invited me to her fine old French colonial house in the middle of the city, where her well-trained servants made excellent martinis and served good food. She drove me about when the occasion arose in her large Mercedes and sometimes on Sundays would invite me to picnics on the beach of a nearby river.

But at the beginning I was naive. Michelle, it became evident, anticipated that our attachment would have its romantic aspects. I was fond of her, and indebted to her, but I failed to hear the music. Aside from that, our relationship was just fine.

Michelle's diplomatic forte was intimate luncheons. These were held at her house, and to them she invited, one at a time, Lao cabinet ministers, generals, ambassadors, and others among the highest-ranking officials. It would seem that none dared refuse her invitations. Sometimes these days, when I watch our television journalists, particularly on those Sunday noon interview programs, I think of Michelle and the sharp, even merciless, fashion in which she questioned luncheon guests. But each invitee appeared to rise to the occasion, and perhaps enjoy it. Certainly each told her more than it would be customary to divulge, and in return each fostered the belief that by doing so he was strengthening his contact with the American embassy.

The problem with this last premise was that Michelle had a very particular point of view on all matters and was often at loggerheads with other, and perhaps prevailing, viewpoints at the embassy.

When I was invited to these luncheon encounters, a privileged third person, I listened, fascinated. My great and special interest in the kingdom was nurtured in this way.

One cabinet minister and former ambassador whom I met at Michelle's table was Nouphat Chounramany, an utterly charming man educated in England. He kept on tap innumerable Lao legends, which he would use to embellish all topics of conversation. He would hold his listeners under his spell. He quickly became a friend and would occasionally invite me to join his wife and family for a meal or a celebration at their comfortable though not lavish home.

Nouphat was also unusual in this kingdom because he was a political chameleon—that is, whichever faction was in charge, he became one of them, whereas most of the other Lao leaders were definitely either in or out of power.

And this brings us to a consideration of the government of Laos.

❋ ❋ ❋

When Laos achieved its independence from the French, it established itself as a constitutional monarchy. The king was a divine figure who lived in his palace in the exquisite northern town of Luang Prabang. The King's Council was there to listen and advise, and His Majesty attended formal functions of state and Buddhist rites. But he insisted that he was not running the government—that was the responsibility of the National Assembly, an elected body, and the prime minister and his cabinet.

All well and good, except that there was three sharply defined political factions that vied for power, and here the story begins to resemble a fairy tale, for each of the three was headed by a prince.

We could say: once upon a time in a tiny kingdom, there were three princes— one was very, very good, and the other two were very, very ambitious. According to my highly subjective point of view, that statement is fairly accurate.

Prince Boun Oum was heir to the former king of Champassak in the southernmost part of the country. Boun Oum was a tall, heavy, outgoing man with a macho charm and an eye for a pretty woman. He looked and acted the celebrity, a Lao version of John Wayne. Although the prince had briefly served as prime minister, he showed little aptitude for political matters other than by encouraging his shrewd and devious protégé, General Phoumi Nosavan. Phoumi had started his career as a noncommissioned officer in the French army and, with the help of family ties to the strongmen of Thailand, had worked his way up through the Lao army. Under the protective cloak of Boun Oum, he was determined to become dictator of Laos. Clever Phoumi saw that his way to success, especially in the presence of the American military, was to proclaim himself the spearhead of the anticommunist forces. He needed no other issues, no other convictions. Human rights could be violated as long as they were violated in the name of anticommunism.

Prince Souphanouvong's father was of the royal Luang Prabang family, but his mother had been a minor wife. Some who knew him well believe that this made him extremely *complexé*—the stepchild who was determined to come out on top. He was certainly intelligent and could be truly charming. While studying in Hanoi, he had married a Vietnamese woman who was a follower of North Vietnam's famous leader, Ho Chi Minh, and she was to be the dominant influence in his life. In the aftermath of the Japanese invasion and departure, Souphanouvong allied himself with North Vietnamese communist elements and proceeded to form a cadre of communist soldiers in Laos. They were called the Pathet Lao, and Souphanouvong became known as the Red Prince.

The third prince was Souvanna Phouma. A cousin of the king and a half-brother of Souphanouvong, he stood directly in the lineage of that branch of the royal family that traditionally governed the kingdom. He was a philosophical man who brought to the country the concept of a neutral nation, one where all Lao could live peacefully and hold free elections.

He was educated in Hanoi and then in France, where he received an engineer's degree from the University of Grenoble and an architect's degree from the University of Paris. When the French retook control of Laos after World War II, he, his wife, and his children went to Bangkok to live in voluntary exile. When the kingdom gained its independence, he returned and served twice as prime minister. But as the rightist forces gained strength and come into power, they wanted him elsewhere, and Prince Souvanna Phouma was appointed ambassador to Paris.

◆ ◆ ◆

When I arrived in Vientiane, Phoumi, with the tacit approval of His Majesty and the encouragement of the American military, was threatening to seize control of a weak government; Souvanna Phouma was still in Paris; and Souphanouvong was in prison in Vientiane, incarcerated by the rightist government.

Souvanna Phouma, Souphanouvong, Boun Oum, and Phoumi Nosavan—these were principal players in the drama of Laos. The Fulbright teacher from New York, through various circumstances in the years that followed, came to know each of them well and within a decade became closely related to two of them.

Let us return to Michelle. She idolized Prince Souvanna Phouma, enjoyed Prince Souphanouvong but deplored his politics, was indifferent to Prince Boun Oum, and detested Phoumi Nosavan.

◆ ◆ ◆

Vientiane was essentially a quiet, informal, tropically green city, but the flame trees which flourished in a row along the river road provided the top of the embankment with a shocking slash of scarlet, and the sunsets across the Mekong were positively majestic in deep orange, burnished red, and magenta, often flecked with slivers of light, bright lime green. A pealing organ would have been the appropriate accompaniment for this evening spectacle.

I liked walking about the town, but then, as far back as I can remember, I have enjoyed walking. When I taught at Hunter and lived in Greenwich Village, most afternoons I covered by foot the sixty blocks from school to the apartment rather than ride.

The river road and the sunset were extraordinary, but even the shops were of interest. They were wide open to the street, secured at night by their metal grilles, through which one could peer if not enter. These stores contained a hodgepodge of merchandise—a single establishment offered such disparate items as oil lamps, electric bulbs, straw matting, bicycles, and whiskey. One rather grand grocery sold only French imports—perfumes, soaps, foie gras, cheeses, wines, and Vichy water. The gold merchants alone had real doors and glass windows in which they displayed chains, bracelets, and rings, all in pure twenty-four–karat, red gold. There was but one bookstore, and its publications were mainly French with some Lao volumes. English was restricted to *Time, Newsweek,* and the *Bangkok Post*. A few eating places served pungent foods ladled out of great pots.

Despite its size and overtones of provincialism, Vientiane gave evidence that it was not a large village but actually a small and cosmopolitan city, quite different from any city I had ever known. In addition to the smiling Lao, the people promenading about represented much of the world and were often readily identifiable. Most were Asians, but there were the French, many of whom wore military uniforms, a good sprinkling of British, a sampling of my fellow Americans, most of them attached to the USAID mission, and, on occasion, a pompously dressed man or couple who would use *nyet* as a negative.

A center of life for the international community was the Hotel Constellation on the main street. Although it was wider than its neighbors and taller—all of four stories high—this concrete building was completely unprepossessing. It, like the stores, opened to the street and was closed at night by its metal grille. On the ground floor it was a bar and cafe with tables to the rear at which meals were served. A simple staircase led up to the three floors of guest accommodations, perhaps twenty rooms in all.

But this was the leading hotel in the city, and almost all of the journalists who were continually checking into and out of Vientiane, whether they were from the East or West, stayed there. The bar and tables near it afforded one of the greatest concentrations of international intrigue since Rick's Cafe in Casablanca.

It seemed to me that each time I went to the Constellation an American intelligence type was there on vigil—and this was understandable. The most obvious of these particular Americans was a Yalesman who affected an accent and manners that were terribly, terribly British. Beneath this off-putting facade, he was a bright and decent fellow who appreciated Prince Souvanna Phouma's efforts and who, unlike too many of his fellow officers, mistrusted Phoumi's facile anticommunism. It was to be expected that he was a good friend of Michelle.

The proprietor of the hotel, our host, was Maurice, a very suave man of Franco-Asian background. He took excellent care of his guests, cashed their checks, arranged their transportation for short or long distances, served them good French food, and all in all made their lives in this city far more comfortable than they would have been without him. A few years later, when the large, river front, government-sponsored Hotel Lan Xang was built, the journalists remained faithful to Maurice.

There were interesting correspondents at the bar of the Constellation. One was a Frenchman whose opinions and writings were sharply pro–Pathet Lao. He was abrasive—and we had several arguments.

Now let us for a moment leap ahead some fifteen years to the evening when he and I ran into each other at a dinner party in Bangkok. I greeted him with reserve, but after the meal, when the women went into the salon and the men into the library, he took me aside and said he wished to speak with me. I listened. Yes, he admitted, he had been procommunist. He blamed what he referred to as his confused idealism that had led him to see this form of socialism as the best solution. Then, after leaving Laos, he had been happy to be posted to Hanoi—that is, happy until he got there. His efforts to talk and reason with Vietnamese officials were in vain. He saw all about him fearful abuses of the civilian population. He found microphones hidden in his hotel room and office, and frequent searches were made of his possessions. He requested an early transfer and left Hanoi as a confirmed anticommunist.

We return to the bar of the Constellation. Another habitué was a somewhat fey and talented British woman, Sarah. Her husband had been in the London theatre, and when she became widowed she came to Asia. She subsisted in Vientiane on a next-to-nonexistent income and inhabited a local brothel/hotel because, as she freely announced, she could not afford to live elsewhere.

But she was an attractive personality who wrote interviews with the leading Lao, and they came to appreciate her. She sent dispatches to top London journals and from time to time would be published. Throughout almost all of my years in Laos, Sarah was there, friendly and amusing and sometimes a source of information.

Flame trees, sunsets, and the characters at the Constellation Bar. These are among my memories of Vientiane.

◆ ◆ ◆

His Majesty King Sisavang Vong died in Luang Prabang in October. He had been ill, and his demise was not unexpected. But Buddhists do not hurry remains to cremation, and the funeral ceremonies for a monarch may be delayed months or years until the auspicious date is determined.

In the meantime the new king, his eldest son, must assume the sovereign functions, although his formal coronation cannot take place until after the funeral of his father. It was still October when I learned quite casually that investiture ceremonies were to be held that very afternoon.

I got on my bike and passed the government circle, in the center of which a lonely cow mooed pathetically. I continued on a road, actually a prolongation of the Avenue Lan Xang but not in any sense comparable to that broad thoroughfare, until it climbed to the wide plateau on which the great Buddhist monument of Tat Luang soars. The Tat is a gilded seventeenth-century *stupa*, unusually and gracefully changing from linear to curved lines as it rises high above a series of brick walls that form a large square enclave. The effect is that of a cloister from the center of which an enormous, eccentric golden tower erupts. Tat Luang is built on the sacred ground where Lord Buddha left his mark.

A hundred or so yards from the enclave is a temple, Wat Hotmam Sapha, which in one major respect does not resemble a temple, for it is an open pavilion, columns without walls. The tall columns, however, sustain a magnificent and traditional temple roof: it swoops down before curving upward, its corners rising into uplifted naga heads.

I left my bicycle against a tree and walked to the pavilion. The royal limousine was nearby, as were other government and diplomatic limousines and autos, but not in any great number. A few royal guards in their resplendent uniforms were in evidence, as were some khaki-clad soldiers. Only the Lao flag, a white three-headed elephant against a red background, served in profusion to announce the event colorfully.

I approached the temple—anyone who wished to could do so. Within were giant silver bowls filled with flowers, and tantalizing Lao music rippled forth from a group of musicians. Mats were spread out on the floor of the temple, and those in attendance sat or reclined on these. To the front of the pavilion His Majesty Savang Vatthana, in a white braided tunic, his legs crossed beneath him, occupied a rug. He was a large man with a large head and sad, sensitive eyes. The queen, crown prince, and other members of the royal family were clustered near him. But also close by were Boy Scouts and young girls, all entirely at their ease. Jacketed members of the diplomatic corps, unused to sitting on a floor for any length of time, tried to give themselves some measure of comfort as they shifted their weight from one buttock to another. And everyone was shoeless, for one does not wear shoes into a Buddhist shrine. Only the presence of a few journalists and photographers was intrusive to this tranquil ritual.

I stood on the side of the temple and watched, as did no more than fifty others. When the music stopped, the *bonzes* chanted and offered prayers and blessings. Then more music, more chanting. The simple ceremony soon arrived at its simple conclusion. The king and queen departed, and the gathering dispersed.

I walked back to my bicycle. I was surprised—surprised by how starkly unaffected the rites had been, surprised that I had been allowed to stand so close as to feel a sense of participation. Had this actually been the investiture of a king? How could this storybook kingdom exist in our times?

◆ ◆ ◆

Living overseas, people of like nationality tend to cling together, except for those few who realize that living abroad offers a rare opportunity for cultural enrichment.

One of the latter was in charge of the USAID health program. He and I had a mutual friend in New York, and I was pleased to be invited to his home for dinner. His other guests were Lao, save for two Indians. These two were night watchmen at the USAID compound, a lowly occupation, but our good host had spoken with them and learned that they were college graduates unable to find work in their own country. They were intelligent and ambitious, and we sympathized with their plight.

Also present was one of the very few Lao physicians. He was worldly and charming, and I was not surprised to learn that he was closely related to the royal family. We became friends. He brought me to his house to meet his wife and children, and on another occasion gave me a tour of the Mahossot Hospital, where he practiced.

He sent me a note one day—I had no telephone—inviting me

to the wedding of a relative, the daughter of a high government official. When he called for me, I with my Western instincts asked if it would be all right for me to go since I had not been formally invited. He laughed.

What we attended, I quickly learned, was not the weddings itself but the reception. Buddhist weddings are intimate family affairs, not a ritual but a richly symbolic ceremony called a *baci*. But their wedding receptions can be just as showy and as extravagant as other peoples'.

This one was held on the lawn of the large family house, with more than a hundred persons gathered beneath red, green, and yellow parachutes spread out and suspended from the trees to offer shelter. The women were magnificent in scarves and skirts of woven silk with borders of gold or silver fabric; the men wore white silk shirts with small standing collars. There were tables and chairs for the guests, several large buffets laden with food and drinks, and a wooden dance platform on which a group of Lao musicians were playing the Lao dance, the *lam vong*.

This was my introduction to the *lam vong*. To perform it, the couple as they reach the dance floor *wai*, or bow, to each other with courtly courtesy and then become part of the circle of dancers, the men outside, the ladies inside. As they dance around the circle, they face each other. Their hands, their marvelously flexible hands, never stop their sinuous motion, but neither do the hands of the couple ever touch each other. The hands bring them together and keep them apart; they say yes, they say no; they invite, they reject. Synchronized with the hand motion is a simple, rhythmic dance step that moves forward and slides backward. The *lam vong* is a moving circle of hands, tenderly, elegantly inviting, then gently, teasingly rejecting. Around and around. The tempo increases. Intoxicating, utterly intoxicating.

It is foolhardy for a foreigner, especially a clumsy Westerner, to attempt this oh so subtle dance. I was given no choice. The doctor had in tow a beautiful young woman in a dazzling silk costume. He presented her and announced that she wished to dance with me. I know this was at his instigation, but there she was, and there was I.

I made a graceless *wai*, and we joined the circle. As we went around, the tempo gradually increasing, I started to lose my sense of conspicuous awkwardness and began to enjoy what I was doing. The more I danced, the more I entered into its spirit. When the young lady left, I found myself *waiing* to other women and going around the circle with them. My hands were in a whirl, while my feet tried to keep the rhythm. I knew I could never hope to bring to this dance the grace I saw all about me, but it ceased to matter. It was such fun. Ever since, I have been an enthusiastic practitioner of the *lam vong* and have sought opportunities to indulge.

Another day, I had another and very different experience with Lao music and dance. I was meandering about the city's own version of Times Square—three large movie houses with loudspeakers blaring surrounded by many foodstands, shops, and more noise. A short distance on was a particularly weatherbeaten barn of a theater with no discernible exterior identification. But walking past, I heard strains of delectable music. I stopped, listened, and tried one of the wooden doors. It was unlocked and I stepped into a stark, rustic auditorium in which rows of benches faced a surprisingly large stage. No one heeded me as I made my way to a bench near the rear of the theater.

The stage door consisted of painted flats, but they were imaginatively done and succeeded in suggesting a fairy-tale forest. The musicians, young boys and men, performed on native instruments: three played simple bamboo flutes, and another three played Pan-like flutes, *khens*, made of bamboo sticks held together by half-gourds from which the mouthpieces protruded. Six musicians bowed two-string violins, two hit xylophone keys strung across wooden boat-shaped boxes, and two other struck cymbals arranged in circular frames that surrounded the players. Muted, exotic music flowed in complete harmony with the stage set—vivid, enticing, exquisite, and unrelated to my world of New York.

The music halted briefly, then resumed. On stage some twenty girls emerged from the wings. They seemed too small and too fragile to support their lavish costumes and headdresses thickly embroidered with heavy gold thread. The girls moved on incredibly supple bare feet, their toes frequently forming graceful arcs. Their bodies were either erect or slightly inclined from the hips— not the waist—a stance which focused attention on their undulating arms and amazing hands, long, thin fingers that curved backward to an implausible degree. Their facial expressions bore a touch of divinity—goddesses with a faint trace of a smile. Their dancing was an extension of the music; it evoked transcendent joy.

The dancers were interrupted several times, for this was a rehearsal, by a gray-haired man who came forward on the stage to change ever so slightly a position or a movement. Then the dance would continue. This I learned was the Ecole Natasinh, the national school of Laos for music and dance.

Many times since, although not nearly as many as I would have wished, I have watched the Lao classic dancers, and each performance has been enchanting.

◆ ◆ ◆

Lao cuisine is unique and delicious but difficult to sample because even in that country restaurants serving it are almost nonexistent. Fortunately, the hospitable Lao readily welcome visitors to their homes and always seem to have more than enough to feed guests.

As is so often the case with regional cuisines, one dish is the star attraction. The Irish have their corned beef and cabbage, the Alsatians *choucroute*, the Belgians *waterzoi*, the Japanese *sushi*, the Thais *tom yam*, and the Lao—they have *khaophoun*.

The family of one of my students kindly invited me to their home for lunch and my first encounter with *khaophoun*. The dish is presented handsomely. Mounds of julienned raw vegetables with their brightly contrasting colors are arranged on a large platter in a manner to delight the eye of any nouvelle cuisine chef. On another platter, thin rice noodles that have been briefly cooked and curled into small portions. When everyone is seated about the table, the noodles are placed in individual bowls and covered with the vegetables. Over these is ladled a thick broth made of fish and pork ground together with coconut milk. It might be mentioned here that in Lao kitchens you will not find oils and butter and cream. Coconut milk replaces them.

Let me admit to my embarrassment that on the day I tasted *khaophoun* I was not happy with the first spoonful. Nor with the second or third. The broth was strong, and my naive palate suspected spoiled fish. In the presence of this most pleasant family who several times asked how I was enjoying the dish, I attempted to be diplomatically evasive, although I was probably too emphatic in the way I rejected the offer of a second helping.

How could I have failed to realize what a rare treat I was experiencing! Today it ranks among my absolutely favorite dishes. Let others sing the glories of bouillabaisse. I'll take my stand for *khaophoun*.

◆ ◆ ◆

Lao names are not easy for Westerners and, therefore, shall not be rattled off in profusion. In this kingdom one is generally known and referred to by his first, not his family name, so for the moment, if the reader can keep in mind the names of the three princes—Souvanna Phouma, Souphanouvong, and Boun Oum—plus that of our heavy, Phoumi Nosavan, that will suffice.

As for most of the others, their names, important though they were to their possessors and to the unfolding of this history, will, to facilitate matters, be identified each time they appear. Thus, when I mention that the prime minister at the time of arrival was Phoui Sananikone, I shall not in future chapters make some reference to Phoui and expect immediate recognition from the reader. Phoui and Phoumi—how easy to confuse. No, if Phoui's name reappears later on, it will bear a tag, such as, Phoui Sananikone, prime minister in 1959.

But now that his name is with us, let us consider the Sananikones.

❋ ❋ ❋

The Sananikones constituted a great mandarin family of the kingdom, and although they were not royal, they thought of themselves as noble enough to rival or surpass Luang Prabang's royalty. Phoui Sananikone was the venerable head of the clan and, yes, in his own terms, an arch rival of Prince Souvanna Phouma. At the end of 1958, he with the assistance of elements of the far right, including Phoumi Nosavan, had been able to oust Souvanna and to replace him as head of the government.

However, Phoui Sananikone was first of all an aristocrat and patriotic Lao. As 1959 rolled on, he found not only that the Vietnamese were strengthening the procommunist Pathet Lao and increasing their own military incursions but that Phoumi Nosavan and his men were making political incursions on his regime.

Phoui Sananikone had at the rightists' urgings placed Prince Souphanouvong in prison in Vientiane and had kept him there, but he resisted Phoumi Nosavan's demands that Souphanouvong be brought to trial as a traitor. Despite their irreconcilable political differences, Phoui Sananikone was far closer socially to Prince Souphanouvong than he was to the upstart Phoumi Nosavan.

At Phoui Sananikone's invitation, United Nations Secretary General Dag Hammarskjold made an official visit to Vientiane in November. This naturally created excitement in diplomatic and government circles, but the population of the city evinced little interest in their distinguished visitor. At the dinner in Hammarskjold's honor, Phoui Sananikone spoke of his "frail, unarmed, and menaced" kingdom. He insisted that Laos must remain neutral and asked the United Nations to support the "efforts of a country toward following its independent path." In short, Phoui Sananikone was committing himself to Souvanna Phouma's attempts at making Laos a neutral, peaceful nation. Hammarskjold listened and appointed a United Nations observer in permanence for the little kingdom.

Phoumi Nosavan, although a cabinet member, was instrumental in forming what he called a Defence Committee for the National Interest. It was made up of the most impatient of the anticommunists and included Khamphan Panya, a keen political manipulator from Luang Prabang whose power stemmed from his personal closeness to King Savang Vatthana, and Sisouk na Champassak, a young and brilliant nephew of Prince Boun Oum. These men liked to be called the Young Turks, but no one was apt to confuse them with young revolutionary liberals.

By mid-December, Phoui Sananikone had lost patience with them. In a totally unexpected action, he ousted Phoumi Nosavan, Khamphan Panya, Sisouk na Champassak, and certain other military figures from his cabinet. The reverberations were great, but the action might have succeeded except that two weeks later the deputy prime minister died, and with his death Phoui Sananikone lost the deputy's constituency and his own control of the National Assembly.

◆ ◆ ◆

The squat National Assembly building on the edge of the government circle housed a series of prolonged sessions. Riding past on my bicycle, I remarked the large number of cars, mostly Mercedes, surrounding it. Inside, the parliamentarians voted to hold new national elections in April and to remain in a legislative capacity until those elections took place. But Phoui Sananikone's efforts to form a new cabinet failed.

The king flew down from Luang Prabang at the end of December and moved into his Vientiane palace on the Mekong in order to confront the government's resignation. The next day, three armored military cars drove up to the palace and stationed themselves in a menacing position. His Majesty forthrightly announced that until such time as a new cabinet was formed, the army was in control of the country's security. The three armored cars had constituted a quiet coup, and what the king did not say, but what this meant, was that the army was in control of the country. This was Phoumi Nosavan's first major triumph. He had been ousted from the government, and so he took over the country.

The Associated Press quoted one of the officials in the prime minister's office as saying: "Please don't dramatize the situation. It's a *coup d'état* Lao style and not on the South American level. It's all *en famille*. No bloodshed."

Any military group planning a coup should be advised that it will inevitably be the subject of a censorious editorial in *The New York Times*. One appeared on January 6 under the heading, "Military Rule in Laos," but its criticism was muted since the junta promised it would hold power only until the king appointed a caretaker government.

His Majesty surely had not read this editorial but on the very next day appointed an interim cabinet under the leadership of another mandarin and former president of the King's Council, Kou Abhay.

The infighting went undercover, and the government could afford to focus on its larger struggle of fending off the Vietnamese.

◆ ◆ ◆

In January, I took advantage of the school holidays to fly to Bangkok, enjoy Singapore, and travel by car up the Malaysian peninsula. I ended the vacation with five days on the island of Penang at a small inn that must have been exactly as it had been when Somerset Maugham frequented the region. It was called the Lone Pine, and its rooms stretched across the beach, each with its wide veranda facing the sea. The water was delicious—fine swimming if you did not get nervous about the rumored sightings of deadly sea serpents. And it was fascinating to watch the fishermen as they hauled in vast nets bulging with flapping catches and to listen to the strange melodies with haunting rhythms that they chanted.

As I walked along the beach, enjoying the sun and the carefree environment, my thoughts frequently raced north to Laos. Although I had spent only a few months in that land, I felt a strong attachment to the little kingdom.

◆ ◆ ◆

The Sunday after I returned to Vientiane, Charlie Searles, Tom, and Evelyn, who made up the American embassy's cultural affairs section, invited me to join them on an outing to Nong Khai in northern Thailand.

It was not exactly easy to reach Nong Khai. We had gone by jeep from Vientiane southeasterly along the river road for some eight miles to the small town of Thadeua. There we had parked the jeep, checked through a Lao customs hut—it was literally a hut—and descended an excessively steep embankment to the river's edge. Here we had to leap upon a *pirogue,* an old narrow boat propelled by a small outboard motor. It was already crowded with passengers, mostly peddlers or farmers engaged in trade on a very small scale. We had to find space on the benches that ran along either side of the boat and then wiggle our behinds onto them. After several efforts, the boat sputtered, fumed, and bumped its way across the mighty Mekong. On the Thai shore we had to make another perilous leap ashore, and Charlie had the misfortune to lose his footing and slip in the mud. He was wearing white trousers. Then we proceeded up an equally steep bank to the Thai customs hut. They checked out our passports and permitted us to enter the city.

Why had we come to Nong Khai? To do a bit of shopping and to have lunch at an undistinguished restaurant. But the real attraction was surely that this offered an excursion into another country.

As we sat eating tasty Thai noodles and shrimp, Charlie spoke about the Lao American Association in Vientiane. This cultural center and school, where hundreds of Lao came to study English, was under Charlie's direction. He told us how he had been able to encourage a group of *bonzes* into enrolling for an English class, and he was now looking for a teacher. It had to be a male teacher for the monks. The class would be held in late afternoons, after *lycée* hours. Would I be interested? I was.

The LAA, as it was always known, employed a system which starts with such basic sentences as: "This is a door," "This is a boy,"

"The boy opens the door," "The boy closes the door." As a class progressed, although vocabulary and structure became complex, the technique remained the same. The system had proven to be effective.

And so one afternoon the following week I stood at the teacher's desk while a dozen *bonzes* in their saffron robes, shaved heads, and sandal-clad or bare feet straggled into the room. A hairless human face, with even the brows shaven, gives strong emphasis to the eyes, and all of those eyes were examining me, some with amusement, some with suspicion. I smiled and tried to make them feel at ease. Some of them smiled back.

We started the lesson, and it was evident that their knowledge of English varied. According to this system, the class should have a uniform knowledge of the language. Therefore, we had to improvise, but we eventually arrived at a method to advance each student's grasp of English.

Those bald heads and searching eyes grew through the next months to be the faces of individuals, as different from each other as were their personalities. For the most part, they were even softer spoken than the students at the *lycée*, but they were interested and serious, and from a teacher's point of view, they offered a rewarding experience.

It would happen from time to time in later years that I would encounter one of them, perhaps walking down a path with his silver begging bowl and black umbrella, and we would exchange greetings. But never did I get to know one of them well, and never did I learn much if anything about his background. This, however, seemed right to me. These were holy men and should be apart as they concentrated on the teachings of Lord Buddha.

◆ ◆ ◆

In New York, for some people, important decisions would be which film to see, which concert to attend, and which new play to purchase seats for immediately. In Vientiane, there were movies being shown, but few, precious few, that one would care to see, and if one longed for a concert or play, one might have to organize it. And one did.

La Société de Mekong was an international group whose *raison d'être* was to produce a few plays each year. It was natural for me to gravitate toward it, as I had done my graduate studies in drama and my thesis on Bernard Shaw. The president of the society was a Lao prince, a fine gentleman who held the meetings at his home. At the first reunion I attended, I learned that the French members were rehearsing a Paris boulevard comedy, *Le Don d'Adele*, but nothing was scheduled in English. At the spur of the moment I offered to direct *Arms and the Man*, and the proposal was just as quickly accepted.

The casting was easy, with several trying out for each role. The assistant cultural attaché, Tom, an alumnus of Princeton's Triangle Club, was a stocky young man who was just right as the Swiss soldier Bluntschli. Madeleine, the British ambassador's beautiful French-English secretary, made the proud maid Louka a wonderfully sensuous creature. For Catherine, Raina's mother, I chose Marga, the Viennese wife of an American officer. Marga was a handsome woman with a strong presence.

With the preliminary runthroughs behind us, we met for our first serious stage rehearsal at the USAID auditorium, where the performances were to be held. The actors were all present with the exception of Marga, and her absence bothered me. I knew she was a very social creature with a calendar crowded with engagements, but I also realized that if we were going to start with absentees we were in trouble. It was time to begin, and I had just asked one of the stage crew to walk through the part of Catherine when bouncing into the auditorium with the vivacity of a Gabor came Marga, announcing that she had been to a cocktail party and would have to go later to a dinner party, but nothing was going to keep her away from a rehearsal. That did it. None of the cast ever missed a rehearsal after that.

Perhaps it was because so little of this type of activity took place in Vientiane that everyone involved brought to his task exceptional energy and enthusiasm. The costumes were intricately designed and painstakingly executed. The sets that filled the stage were handsome, and a former stage electrician now working with USAID lighted them professionally, even though he was severely limited as to equipment.

We scheduled two performances, both for the benefit of the Red Cross. They sold out well in advance with many Lao dignitaries and members of the diplomatic corps among the ticket holders.

I had personally supervised the program's cover, title page, and credits, but putting together the program was the responsibility of a bright young Lao in the administrative section of the embassy. He kept assuring us that the program would be printed on time and would be full of paid advertisements, which would add considerably to our intake.

An hour before curtain time, the programs were delivered to the auditorium, and they looked very good indeed. As I scanned through one, I arrived at a certain page and my head must have snapped back. It was a full page displaying the photo of a man, naked except for a very small strategically placed cloth, stretched out on a table. Hovering above him was a scantily clad lass. The wording beneath was restrained: "Relaxing, refreshing, White Rose." Our eager entrepreneur in charge of the program had sold the space to the White Rose Massage Parlor. Prude that I was, my first reaction was to have that page torn out of each program, but on second thought, this was not only foolish but also destructive, for a list of credits for the play appeared on the other side of that page. Therefore, the programs were distributed to the members of the audience as they arrived.

The Lao, as I mentioned, are a spirited people, and they, I suspect, were amused by the program. The play went off splendidly, except that some of Shaw's piquant remarks about society and war in Bulgaria sounded as though they might pertain to society and war in the little kingdom. But no protests were voiced.

* * *

Here come the clowns. But these are not comedians who evoke laughter. These are fearfully greedy men whose leader, Phoumi Nosavan, will not only hasten the downfall of the little kingdom but will try to destroy its gentle nature. And it pains me to note that these clowns will be strongly encouraged by many, although by no means all, elements of the American mission.

The cabinet set up in January 1960 under Kou Abhay was dominated by the members of the Defense Committee for the National Interest, the very persons whom the moderate Prime Minister Phoui Sananikone had had good reason to oust from his government. This cabinet was identified as a caretaker government whose main task was to prepare for national elections in April. Nothing in the conduct of these rightists was more efficient than the preparation for those elections. They went to extremes to make certain that the balloting would be rigged in their favor.

The atmosphere started to turn sour during this period. Previously, the struggle between communists and anticommunists had been to a large measure a family affair, and each side had maintained that its victory could best guarantee a continuation of the kingdom's gentle way of life. Political assassinations and bloodshed had been rare.

◆ ◆ ◆

It so happened that directly across the street from my lodgings was a government building which had once been a school and which now was used, it was said, for certain administrative purposes. It was not much of a building and was not well maintained. Nevertheless, there was some vaguely sinister air about it, especially a ground floor area where the windows were barred and darkly curtained and where soldiers often loitered.

A European-educated Lao acquaintance who, I knew from conversations, had no fondness for the present government, came by one day, and I asked him casually about the building across the street. He regarded me curiously and demanded to know why I was asking. With no good reason to offer, I was ready to drop the subject. But he was not. He hesitated and then explained some facts of Laos to me.

The ground floor area was, he told me, a prison of sorts. This was the private security quarters of Colonel Siho, General Phoumi's closest and most feared aide. The colonel was known to bring those whom he considered to be dangerous adversaries of Phoumi or himself into these quarters, to confine them there, to torture them, to maim them, and sometimes to murder them.

I do not know the truth of these accusations against Colonel Siho, although later I was to hear them repeated by some highly reputable sources. However, the very existence of such charges reveals far too much about the natures of both Siho and his mentor, and about the extent to which the gentle traditions of the kingdom were being destroyed.

◆ ◆ ◆

Before the elections in April, I joined Charlie, Tom, and Evelyn for a weekend at Phou Khao Kwai, a government rest house in the mountains some fifty miles north of Vientiane where Charlie had reserved rooms for us. We bounced for hours as the jeep struggled over a rock-strewn road. But as we climbed, the dusty heat of the city fell behind, and we entered an inviting mountain forest. We forded rivulets, passed hill tribe villages, and at last reached the rustic inn. It had a thatched roof, four guest bedrooms, and a veranda. The toilet and shower were underneath the structure.

The inn possessed a special grand attraction: the proprietress was a French-Hungarian woman who was a splendid chef. She prepared delectable meals with a heavy Hungarian flavor. To eat this way in the mountains of Laos was totally unexpected and incredibly pleasurable.

We meandered about the area and visited the nearest village, where the houses, in traditional fashion, were on stilts. The villagers in their colorful costumes were neither accommodating nor unfriendly; they maintained a dignified air. Not too far from the inn, I found a natural pool and was happy to take off my clothes and jump into the water. Mountain lakes always delight me.

In the evening we were joined by another guest, a Frenchman from Vientiane who was searching for additions to his important collection of wild orchids. And he was finding them.

The visit passed quickly, and on Sunday afternoon we left this delightful mountain retreat to drive back to the civilization of Vientiane.

Sadly, the experience remains especially memorable for an appalling reason. The atmosphere of the kingdom under confrontational circumstances had been growing tense. The very weekend after our excursion, a French educator temporarily affiliated with the Lao Ministry of Education went to Phou Khao Kwai with his wife and two children. In the morning, some fifty tribesmen arrived on the scene, surrounded the inn, and demanded that the occupants come out. The Frenchman walked out to speak to them, and they slew him. They then took his wife and the proprietress, tied their arms behind their backs, and marched them off into the hills. The desperate wife was able to communicate with a leader of the group. He informed her that they were pro–Pathet Lao and were doing this to wreak vengeance on the Americans. The wife after some hysterical arguing convinced him that she and the innkeeper were French, not Americans. The two women were released.

The rest house was, of course, closed as of that day. The French ambassador in Vientiane was kind and clever enough to offer refuge to the innkeeper, who became a stellar addition to his kitchen.

I cannot forget that those Pathet Lao–inspired tribesmen had been seeking Americans as a target for death, and we had been the last Americans at Phou Khao Kwai.

❊ ❊ ❊

Phoumi Nosavan's extreme right-wing party declared itself winner of all fifty-nine seats in the new National Assembly. His colleague, Khamphan Panya, rejoiced in the results and vociferously denied that left-wing voters had been subjected to pressures or that the results had been tampered with.

That was not the way others viewed the election results. On May 1, Jacques Nevard, *The New York Times* correspondent, wrote from Vientiane:

> If the election results were to be taken at face value, they would show that Laos, which had been heavily infiltrated by communists from neighboring communist North Vietnam, had resoundingly repudiated pro-communist candidates. The fact, however, is that almost no one had any faith in the returns, which included lop-sided victories for army-backed right-wing candidates in strongly communist districts.
>
> The big question in Laos is: what are the communists going to do about it? Most observers think that the communists, having sought a voice in the government by democratic means and having been thwarted, might well abandon the idea of a political solution and concentrate on a military one.

Nevard knew Laos well, but no one could have predicted the events that turned the kingdom topsy-turvy in the following months.

A lovely bit of comedy occurred in late May. Prince Souphanouvong and a group of his followers, some fifteen in all, were still incarcerated in the Vientiane prison, but one night someone opened the jail cells, and the Red Prince and his followers escaped into the jungle. They decidedly had no intention of allowing themselves to be dealt with by this new Phoumi government. Souphanouvong was next heard from up in northern Pathet Lao territory.

◆ ◆ ◆

Something also happened to me. The United States Information Agency had sent out a team from Washington to give the Vientiane post its biannual inspection. The team was there for several weeks, and before it left its chief summoned me to his office. He told me he thought I had the makings of a good foreign service officer and that if I wished he would recommend me for such an appointment. I had no hesitation in replying: Yes, I would like to be in the Foreign Service.

Shortly thereafter, with the school year ended and with General Phoumi blatantly if not firmly in command of the government, I took my departure from the little kingdom and headed back to New York.

❅ ❅ ❅

That summer of 1960 when I left Vientiane to return to New York and my teaching chores at Hunter College, the Lao government was the darling of the Americans. Prince Somsanith was the prime minister, and he was a quiet, plodding, but wholly respectable member of the nobility who, if asked, would say softly that his was a neutral government. But it was not. The man in power was General Phoumi Nosavan. From within the tiny kingdom, Phoumi kept rattling American-provided swords against the communists, and the Americans, in gratitude, increased their support. This support became more than generous: it became overwhelming. Every soldier in the Royal Lao Army received his salary from United States funds.

Prince Souvanna Phouma had returned from his Paris ambassadorship to resume a leading role in the National Assembly and to attempt to bring some moderation to the government. And Prince Souphanouvong was up in the northern provinces, where the Pathet Lao and the North Vietnamese continued to advance their invasion of the land.

Then everything changed. On August 9, there occurred in the city one of the most remarkable *coup d'états* in modern history. But to tell how it came about, a nursery rhyme rephrased seems most apropos:

> Phoumi, Phoumi, where have you been?
> I've been to Luang Prabang to visit the king.

And so he had. General Phoumi with most of his closest officers went to call on His Majesty. During the night of his absence, a young paratroop captain by the name of Kong Le sent his forces, small in number, throughout the city. With virtually no opposition, they took over the government buildings, radio stations, and barracks and proclaimed a new government.

One's reaction is apt to be: Well, what makes this such a remarkable coup? It sounds conventional. But it wasn't. Young Captain Kong Le at once announced his goals: Lao must stop fighting Lao, and the kingdom must be independent and neutral.

Yet, you may say, many a military leader speaks this way upon achieving his coup, but this is almost invariably a prelude to the leader's decision that the only person capable of bringing his country to the desired position is himself. That was not true for Kong Le.

Who was this captain? He was short and slight of build and sometimes wore a shy smile. He came from a hill tribe family, attended the *lycée* of Vientiane, entered the army, and received paratroop training in Thailand and the Philippines. His knowledge of French and English was good, but he was reticent to speak them. It has always been difficult to pin down his age, but at the time of the coup he was in his late twenties or early thirties. He was set apart from the rank and file by having married the daughter of a prominent Lao general, but his life-style was simple. He had no auto and managed to get around Vientiane on a bicycle.

Many members of the American community were surprised, and disappointed, that the people of Vientiane so cheerfully accepted the advent of a new government and the sudden departure of General Phoumi, Colonel Siho, and their cohorts. Kong Le became the people's instant and authentic hero.

Three days after the coup, he announced a political rally at the National Stadium. To call this small athletic field, with a dozen rows of bleacher benches along one side, a National Stadium sounds pretentious, but so be it. On the given evening, the normally undemonstrative people of the city were exuberant, and they came in a great outpouring to the field. While waiting, musicians played the *khens* and singers and dancers performed. When Kong Le, still in a simple khaki uniform, arrived in a jeep, he received a deafening ovation. "Kong Le, Kong Le, Kong Le," they chanted.

When he managed to silence the crowd, he addressed them as a simple man, not as a conqueror or orator. His speech was delivered without notes, and the phrasing was often hesitant, but the message came through clearly.

He denounced the government of Somsanith—it was bellicose and dishonest. He decried continuation of the fighting that had pitted Lao against Lao. "We are tired," he said, "of civil wars." He declared that if such a war persisted, it would destroy the country and the people.

His was a plea for neutrality. He stated: "We will incline neither to the free world nor to the communist world." Oh, brave young captain! He underscored the statement by adding: "We will accept diplomatic relations with all countries." One can imagine the shudder that went through the American community upon hearing this pronouncement.

He continued: "The government of Prince Somsanith must resign. Laos needs at its head a leader who is strong and honest, and one who has already proven himself. There is such a leader," the captain asserted, "one who will unite the country in strength and neutrality, and that leader is Prince Souvanna Phouma."

Remarkable coup! The young military rebel took over the government not to gain glory for himself but to save his country. He asked no role for himself. He wanted the leadership to go to a man he hardly knew on a personal basis, but a man he respected and admired.

It is puzzling to know what in Kong Le's relatively simple background had propelled him into this extraordinary act of patriotism.

As in much of the story of Laos, there are comic elements. The *coup d'état* caught Prince Souvanna completely by surprise. He promptly declared that he had nothing to do with these rebels, and furthermore wanted nothing to do with them. After several days of persuasion, the prince accepted the position he was being offered. When the National Assembly met, the building was completely ringed by Captain Kong Le's tanks and soldiers. Under these circumstances, it was not surprising that the members of the Assembly voted with unanimity to disband Prince Somsanith's government and to replace it with a new one headed by Prince Souvanna Phouma. Their decision was sent to the king in Luang Prabang, who, after some hesitation, and with some reluctance, acceded to the Assembly's demand.

Within a week, the country had a new government with Prince Souvanna as prime minister. But this new government became almost at once the target of a barrage of attacks from both inside and outside the country. These took the form of military, economic, and psychological onslaughts. The enemies were the right-wing Lao, the Pathet Lao, the North Vietnamese, Thailand, and, most devastatingly, the United States.

◆ ◆ ◆

General Phoumi Nosavan liked to receive his visitors on the veranda of his large modern house on the outskirts of Savannakhet. From the veranda, a wide green lawn extended down to the Mekong. The setting was deceptively calm and peaceful.

The general was stocky, and his face, well suited to his frame, was heavy and squarish. He looked at people penetratingly, but not receptively. He smiled infrequently, and the smile, when it appeared, lacked mirth. When life went well for him—as it seemed to do shortly after the coup—his visage wore an especially smug expression.

Savannakhet, a city southeast of Vientiane, had in recent years become a realm over which he held sway. It was also southern headquarters for the army, and after the little captain had ousted him from the capital, Phoumi quickly amassed in this city a large part of what had been the Royal Lao Army.

The general spent much time at the army base, where the activity was accelerated. Not only were soldiers who had defected from the new government arriving in numbers, but quite a few Americans could be found here. They were members of the military and intelligence who had come to oversee the training of Phoumi's army, to equip the soldiers, and to render them the invincible force of the kingdom. It did not matter to these Americans that the United States embassy pretended to support the official government in Vientiane.

In late afternoon, on his veranda, Phoumi would occasionally offer drinks to some of his aides and to some of the Americans. Once in a while Prince Boun Oum would come up from his fief of Champassak to join them. The fiction was that Boun Oum was the mentor, but of course it was the protégé who was completely in charge.

Urgent messages arrived from Vientiane. The prime minister wanted the general to meet with him in either Luang Prabang or Vientiane to try to resolve the problems of the divided country. Phoumi naturally declined these invitations, for he knew that time and the Americans were on his side.

It encouraged him to look across the river to Thailand—so close by, and so convenient for bringing in supplies about which Vientiane could remain ignorant. Phoumi's relations with this neighboring country were excellent. Sarit Thanarat, Thailand's head of government, was distantly related but closely allied. Sarit's ruthless rise to power through the Thai military ranks served as an inspiration to the Lao general.

* * *

In September, only a month after the coup, intelligence reports confirmed that Pathet Lao–North Vietnamese troops were posing a threat to a northern Lao province. Souvanna Phouma planned to send assistance to help defend the province's capital, Samneua. But Phoumi and his American aides wanted to take this on for the Savannakhet team. Phoumi therefore quickly sent five hundred of his men to safeguard Samneua and spurned Souvanna's offer of cooperation. To help his ally, Sarit entered into the fray. Since all of Vientiane's supplies, vital and otherwise, had to reach the inland city through Thailand, Sarit instituted an unofficial but effective blockade. Commodities became scarce in the kingdom's capital.

An as though that were not enough, some shells were fired from the Thai side of the Mekong and exploded in Vientiane. In that city, one could not be certain whether these had been fired by elements of the Pathet Lao, or by Phoumi's men, or by the Thai, but Prince Souvanna Phouma declared that he was holding the Thai government accountable for these attacks. The shelling stopped.

Convinced that he could now take on the government army, General Phoumi Nosavan sent twelve hundred men as the advance for his plan to attack and capture Vientiane. As Phoumi's soldiers were on their way north and approached the town of Paksane, they were surprised by Kong Le and two hundred of his lightly equipped men. The little captain routed the right-wing army, and Phoumi's troop fled, leaving behind machine guns, rifles, and mortars.

Shortly thereafter Samneua fell to the leftists.

And so General Phoumi suffered two notable defeats—by Kong Le at Paksane, and by the Pathet Lao at Samneua. And yet the general did not seem discouraged. Standing on the veranda, looking out over the Mekong, with Prince Boun Oum beside him, he boasted that soon Vientiane would be his.

* * *

On the first day of October, Prince Souvanna Phouma in a radio address to his countrymen told them that communism destroys Buddhism. "I assure you," he promised, "I shall not allow communism to rule our country." He continued by saying that although he would respect communism in those countries in which it had been established, "we only ask them not to try to spread their doctrine—which opposes our religion and traditions—into this kingdom." Despite the clarity and sincerity of this message, some of the Americans involved in Laos remained suspicious because it was not, according to them, sufficiently anticommunist.

The American financing of the kingdom reached an absurd dilemma. Forty million dollars a year was being spent to pay the Lao soldiers, but now that the soldiers were divided among the neutralist and the rightists, what was to be done? The United States wavered about these payments to the government in Vientiane but not about the unofficial large payments that flowed into Savannakhet. But when we put on our most formal, official hat, we did this: the full army payment was made to the treasurer in Vientiane, and an agent from Savannakhet was there to collect from him the rebel's fair share.

The American who led the official opposition to neutralism and to Souvanna Phouma was J. Graham Parsons. A New Englander with a standoffish personality, he had had no difficulty in resisting the warmth and charm of Southeast Asia. And he was rigid in his convictions. For him, the idea of neutralism was synonymous with anti-Americanism, and since Souvanna Phouma was the author of neutralism for Laos, for Parsons the prince was the villain.

J. Graham Parsons had served as ambassador to Vientiane in 1958 and had certainly been involved in the internal maneuverings that had gone on during that period. These included unseating then prime minister Souvanna Phouma, replacing him with the government of Phoui Sananikone, and arranging for the prince to be sent overseas as ambassador to Paris.

Back in Washington, Graham Parsons was rewarded by being made assistant secretary of state. In the autumn of 1960, when Souvanna Phouma's neutralist government was trying to strengthen itself, Parsons took it upon himself to return to Vientiane on an official visit so that he could once again exert his influence to undermine Prince Souvanna in favor of General Phoumi.

The assistant secretary met twice with the prime minister, although they did not break bread together. With the apparent belief that the head of the government of this little kingdom needed some lessons in the way of the world, Parsons lectured him. Prince Souvanna never enjoyed being lectured. Among his remarks, Parsons warned that the communists "did not play a neutral game" and that if the prince wished to be neutral, he would surely eventually be disillusioned. The assistant secretary denied to the press that he was interfering in the internal affairs of another country and seemingly saw no arrogance in trying to force his simplistic Phoumi-style anticommunism upon the foremost proponent of neutralism in Southeast Asia.

Prince Souvanna Phouma had always declared that his government would welcome all factions—Kong Le's coup and the resulting administration were based on that premise. By what may be termed a mischievous coincidence, the official opening of relations with the Soviets took place in October while Parsons was there. The first Soviet ambassador to Laos arrived at Wat Tay and was met at the airport by a crowd of well-wishers led by Kong Le. The little captain offered the envoy an overly enthusiastic reception, for which he was reprimanded by the prime minister.

Parsons, furious, made a swift and ungracious departure. The Soviet ambassador snidely remarked that he would have liked to have met Mr. Parsons and that it was too bad he had left in such a hurry.

❋ ❋ ❋

At the end of October, all confrontational activities came to a sudden halt. It was the beginning of the annual Tat Luang festival. Asked what would happen should a new crisis arise during this period, Prince Souvanna replied, "But nothing will happen. After all, this is Tat Luang." And the celebration went on unmarred.

However, in November the war grew uglier. Government forces in Luang Prabang defected to Phoumi Nosavan's army.

The prime minister was queried by journalists about a possible settlement of this internal warfare. He said sadly: "It all depends on the Americans." The next day he expanded his comment to declare gravely that the United States was illegally supporting Phoumi Nosavan's war efforts.

British, French, and other foreign diplomats were quoted by the Associated Press as saying that the Americans had thrust Souvanna Phouma into the waiting arms of the communists. The diplomats were wrong. Souvanna Phouma had been pushed by Americans toward the communists, but the prince remained his own man.

In December, with a large Phoumi army making its way north toward Vientiane and with the Pathet Lao forces demanding to take over Kong Le's small and imperiled army, Prince Souvanna Phouma realized that his urgent, desperate appeals for peace were being ignored. About to be crushed between the American-backed troops of the right and the North Vietnamese strength of the left, he stated that he could no longer govern the kingdom.

The prince left for Cambodia.

❀ ❀ ❀

Now comes an appalling event, an utter tragedy. In December, General Phoumi Nosavan's forces made their long-threatened attack upon Vientiane. They arrived this time in large numbers and well supplied with tanks and heavy armament. One need not ask where this equipment came from.

Kong Le prepared his army for the defence of the city, and accepted North Vietnamese–Pathet Lao assistance.

It was indecent and outrageous for Phoumi to ravage this civilian city, but should Kong Le have chosen to defend Vientiane at what was certain to be an enormous loss of life and property?

The battle raged for three days. To distinguish the attackers from the attacked, the former wore white armbands, the latter red armbands. As the armies charged up the streets and then often back in retreat, the terrorized civilians improvised their own white and red armbands and changed them in accordance with whichever army was in the vicinity.

Whatever the civilians did, they were of course the losers. Conflagration swept through many of the poor parts of the city. The Mahossot Hospital, filled with sick and wounded, was shelled. Hundreds perished and innumerable others were wounded.

The American embassy, in which the entire American staff was sequestered for the three days, received a direct mortar hit, which knocked down a wall.

And this took place in a quiet city of gentle people. Phoumi Nosavan's forces prevailed. The battle afforded Western journalists what they deemed to be a clarification of the Lao situation. Without exception, they declared that the neutralist forces had united with the communist forces—perhaps because of those red armbands. That, however, is not what had happened. Kong Le and his men regrouped at new headquarters on the northern plains. This was Pathet Lao territory, but Kong Le made very sure that his army kept apart from the Pathet Lao army.

* * *

Prince Souvanna Phouma spent weeks in Phnom Penh as the guest of his friend and sometime political sparring partner, Prince Sihanouk. *Time* magazine in its Asian edition did a cover story on these two national leaders, the Lao trying to maintain his country's independence through his skills as a statesman, the Cambodian seeking the same goal for his country by means of his flamboyant appeals and prima donna personality.

Souvanna Phouma was extraordinary. He was elegant without affectation, an intellectual who expressed himself simply and directly. His was a commanding presence, and he was both exigent and kind. His moral standards were exceptionally high, not sanctimonious. As a devout Buddhist, he was tolerant to a rare degree. He was respected and admired by his own countrymen and by diplomats throughout the world. His opponents feared him because he acted on his convictions and could not be motivated by ambition or greed. His servants were devoted to him.

Of medium height and slightly heavy, he had as his most striking feature heavy dark eyebrows. His facial expression was friendly and composed, except on those infrequent occasions when he allowed his temper to show.

Whether presiding over affairs of state or playing the social host, he was at ease and intrinsically courteous. He was a superb bridge player and had enjoyed his tennis until, in his seventies, he had to give it up for reasons of health. He was also an ardent gardener.

One day in January, a reporter for *The New York Times*, eager for an interview, went to Phnom Penh to a guest house of Sihanouk in which Souvanna was temporarily residing. The journalist found the prince in the garden, vigorously pruning trees and bushes. As the interviewer posed his questions, the prince continued his horticultural endeavors, as though strenuous exercise would help stem the anger he felt over recent events.

He dismissed Boun Oum and Phoumi Nosavan as fools and incompetents, but he kept his strongest words for J. Graham Parsons. The prince declared: "He [Parsons] understood nothing about Asia, and nothing about Laos. . . . He is the ignominious architect of disastrous American policy toward Laos. He and others like him are directly responsible for the recent spilling of Lao blood."

The report of this interview in a Cambodia garden was a front-page story in *The New York Times* of January 20, 1961.

Within days after this, Prince Souvanna Phouma left Cambodia to join the neutralist army on the plains of Laos and to strengthen that army's resolve against uniting with the Pathet Lao.

The horrendous battle had brought Phoumi Nosavan and his army to Vientiane, but the tiny kingdom remained at war, a three-sided war with the factions headed by Boun Oum, Souvanna Phouma, and Souphanouvong.

◆ ◆ ◆

How incongruous! Here in the latter part of the twentieth century we have what might be termed the War of the Three Princes.

◆ ◆ ◆

While these events were taking place in Laos, I was teaching at Hunter, reading every scrap of news I could find about the little kingdom, and waiting impatiently to hear word on my government application.

In September of 1960 I was again summoned to Washington, this time for an interview, but an interview unlike any I had previously experienced. I was grilled for three hours by a panel of five foreign service officers. They were impressive. One asked probing questions about American policy on China. Although my views differed markedly from those of the administration, I did not attempt to modify them; I suspected these panel members would have seen through any evasion on my part. Another man queried me on American literature and brought up minor early writers whom I had imagined only another teacher of the subject would be likely to know. Two asked about aspects of domestic and international economy—there I was weak. At the conclusion of the long, long session, I had no doubt but that these five inquisitors were in position to judge whether or not I should become a colleague. I was delighted to learn of their affirmative report.

There was one more hurdle. This was the period—and it lasted only briefly—when the State Department was having all potential foreign service officers checked out by psychiatrists. I was assigned to a distinguished doctor of French background and was scheduled for several hours with him. We immediately got on the subject of Stendhal and spent most of the allotted time on French literature. This was in October, during the presidential campaign. Near the conclusion of our last session, the psychiatrist remarked that we had been discussing almost exclusively things I liked.

"Tell me," he said, "what do you dislike?"

From the top of my head came the instant reply: "Richard Nixon."

He laughed heartily, stopped suddenly, and solemnly intoned: "That was a foolish answer. Suppose I were a Republican?"

Word came in January that I was to go to Washington to be sworn in.

* * *

The Boun Oum–Phoumi Nosavan government was in difficulty from its inception. An unpleasant change took place in Vientiane, where the quality of life deteriorated rapidly. In a city in which unlocked front doors had been customary, burglaries suddenly became commonplace. Gambling rooms proliferated. A school building located on the road to Wat Tay airport was converted under quasi-government auspices into a large gambling casino. In the countryside, fighting continued, and government spokesmen issued conflicting claims of military victories or communist attacks.

Time magazine in the last week of January was banned in the kingdom. In it an article on Laos told of "the spectacle of one pro-communist captain with a nucleus of 300 paratroopers standing off a 29,000-man army nurtured and trained by the United States." Twenty-nine thousand seems perhaps too large a number, and certainly Kong Le should have been referred to as antirightist rather than procommunist, but the essence of the statement is irrefutable: General Phoumi, with all of his American support, was an utterly incompetent would-be Napoleon.

Prince Souvanna Phouma, impatient for results, left the plains and traveled throughout Asia and Europe to enlist support for the neutralist cause. While at a dinner party in Florence, an Italian countess was presented to him. Thrilled to be meeting this member of Asian royalty, she asked what for her was an important question: "*Altezza*, in what style is your palace?"

"Madame," the prince replied, "in the style of a military tent."

Phoumi Nosavan's army embarked on a major project: to clear the road between Vientiane and the royal capital of Luang Prabang, one hundred and fifty miles to the north. By the middle of March, the army had succeeded in advancing no further than Vang Vieng, a town some sixty miles north of Vientiane. A small group of Kong Le's men in a brilliant surprise maneuver attacked, and Phoumi's troop fled in panic.

This was the turning point. The new government which three months earlier had battled its way into power, which had proclaimed itself proudly and arrogantly, was reduced to a humiliating posture. Phoumi was forced to seek a defensive cease-fire.

* * *

John Kennedy became president, and that event had a profound effect upon the little kingdom halfway around the earth. The new president proved from the start that he had been studying the situation and declared that the United States favored a neutral Laos, in direct contradiction to Mr. Parsons's position. And the president did more than make statements. He quickly sent his finest envoy, Governor Averell Harriman, to Asia to do an on-site study of the predicament and to advise the White House.

While the governor was in Delhi with Prime Minister Nehru, he met Prince

Souvanna Phouma. The meeting between Harriman and Souvanna was momentous. The two statesmen formed a friendship—a true friendship, not an acquaintanceship—that was to last throughout their lifetimes.

◆ ◆ ◆

Let me digress for a moment to remark that accompanying the prince was his daughter, Princess Moune. Having completed her studies at the Institute of Political Science and the School of Oriental Languages in Paris, she was devoted to her father and to her country. In recent years, on two occasions, the ever debonair Harriman told me that her presence at this initial meeting led him to the conclusion that "any man who had a daughter like Moune must be all right."

✳ ✳ ✳

During this springtime, it was proposed that a new international conference be held in Geneva to resolve the Lao situation. The Geneva conference on Indochina in 1954 could hardly be called a success, but many believed that another try should be made. Prime Minister Nehru and Prince Sihanouk were among the diligent advocates, and the communist powers, for reasons of their own, supported the suggestion. The Harriman–Souvanna Phouma meeting in Delhi advanced the prospects.

Months of negotiations to get the conference organized followed. Finally details seemed in place, but on the day before the official opening, an argument about seating almost unhinged it.

At last, on May 16, 1961, the International Conference on the Settlement of the Laotian Question, as it was formally called, opened in Geneva. The two chair countries were Great Britain and the Soviet Union. The others of the fourteen-nation parley were Burma, Cambodia, Canada, China, France, India, Poland, Thailand, North Vietnam, South Vietnam, and the United States. Laos itself had three opposing delegations, representing Princes Souvanna Phouma, Boun Oum, and Souphanouvong. The conference met, according to the convocation, because "there exist real conditions for the normalization of the situation" in Laos.

And so it came to pass that in the year 1961 the mightiest powers of this globe assembled to argue at great length the future of the little kingdom.

II

Down Then Up the Mekong

1961–1963

T he pompous palace is haunted by the ghosts of the League of Nations. It reeks of the past—is out of place in the present. The United Nations personnel who work there know that they really do not belong in this deceased monument so magnificently set on the shores of Lac Leman in Geneva.

In its vast meeting rooms late in the spring of 1961, teams representing the thirteen nations and the three Lao factions began the task of trying to solve the political problems of the little kingdom, a task that would go on for fifteen months. The conferees argued, went around and around in circular elocutions. They met, recessed, met again, recessed again. But the spirit of Laos was present, and so after hours, the fiercest of opponents would have drinks together, dine together, play tennis together.

The permanent representatives stayed on and on, or were replaced by fellow countrymen. The celebrities came and went. Sir Malcolm MacDonald of Great Britain was the cochair of the conference. Averell Harriman headed the American delegation until he was called back to Washington to become assistant secretary of state, but even in that imposing role he found time and reason to return to the gathering in Geneva. Prince Sihanouk rented a lakefront chalet in which he entertained at dinner parties those he sought to influence. And Krishna Menon, the celebrated Indian firebird, dashed in and out as he planned, plotted, and intrigued to have the conference adopt a resolution with which his country could be comfortable.

The thirteen nations quickly, albeit unofficially, separated themselves into three groups, each offering its support to a different Lao prince. The small nations of Southeast Asia tended to be in Boun Oum's camp. Fearful of a communist invasion, Thailand, the Philippines, and South Vietnam had been against the very concept of another Geneva conference. They wanted Phoumi Nosavan to continue as the power in Vientiane, and although they could hardly announce it, they were almost certainly delighted to have negotiations drag on with little progress month after month.

The communist countries represented in Geneva were the natural allies of Prince Souphanouvong and the Pathet Lao. They, however, realized that a Lao government headed by Souphanouvong would be unacceptable to the majority of the nations and to the other two Lao delegations. For them, nothing would be worse than having the little kingdom continue to be ruled by the Boun Oum–Phoumi Nosavan clique. Therefore, they were willing to accept a government headed by Prince Souvanna Phouma, but they insistently attached impediments to the ongoing arguments and added complications to the ultimate resolution in order to weaken the new government's potential strength.

For France, Great Britain, India, and Canada, for Prince Sihanouk's Cambodia and President Kennedy's United States, it was vital that this vulnerable and strategically located kingdom be neutral. They wanted it to be a zone of truce, of peace if possible, forming a line of demarcation for the communists in that part of the world. They firmly supported a government headed by Souvanna Phouma.

Among the Lao delegations, Boun Oum's was the largest and included such members of the mandarin families as former Prime Minister Phoui Sananikone—despite the altercations he had had with Phoumi Nosavan—Phoui's younger brother, the jovial Ngon Sananikone, and wealthy, stodgy Pheng Norindr—who both earlier and later was a neutralist. Also in this camp were former ambassador Nouphat and those two fellow rebels of Phoumi Nosavan, Khamphan Panya of Luang Prabang and Sisouk na Champassak, nephew of Boun Oum.

Head of the neutralist delegation was Quinim Polsena a rather unpleasant man, but his fellow delegates included the splendid young intellectual Khamchan Pradith and Pheng Norindr's capable and witty bother La Norindr. Princess Moune Souvanna Phouma also served for the neutralists.

The intelligent and often genial Phoumi Vongvichit was spokesman for the Pathet Lao delegation. He later became interim president of the People's Republic of Laos.

One of the early resolutions adopted at Geneva proclaimed that the Lao were to form their own coalition government and choose their own prime minister. As has been mentioned, each of the thirteen nations had his preferred prince, but this method of proceeding gave the conference a seemingly democratic cloak. It would also mean that when matters did not work out, one could say the Lao had only themselves to blame. And so during the fifteen months, while the nations argued in the palace in Geneva, the more important activity took place away from Geneva each time the three princes got together.

Most of us have some idea as to the problems of arranging a summit meeting between heads of state, especially when the states are of unfriendly ideologies. We have an inkling of the enormous jockeying that goes on to decide upon conditions, agenda, location, and so forth. To get our three princes of Laos together for an official meeting seemed no less difficult. After all, these three were rivals and had been in combat. But the pressure coming from Geneva prevailed.

In June, the princes met in Switzerland, but not in Geneva. They gathered in Zurich, and this was one of the more promising of their sessions, for here they announced their intention to form a government of national union.

As unintentional evidence of just how cosmopolitan they were, while the June meeting was held in the ultrasophisticated city of Zurich, their next gathering, in October, took place in Hin Heup in the remote bush area of Laos. A tent was set up on an old war-scarred wooden bridge that crossed a river which sometimes marked a separation between the rightist and communist areas. They met in the tent.

On the first day, the three princes were together for five hours, and the media people who had gathered on the south, or rightist, bank of the river were informed as the participants left the tent that no announcements were forthcoming. The next day, the three principals, or princes if one wishes, delegated three representatives to *pourparler* in the tent. On the third day, our princes returned to huddle inside the canvas for four hours. At the conclusion of this session, a broadly smiling Prince Souvanna Phouma emerged and crossed the bridge to speak to the waiting journalists and photographers. He announced that a final accord had been reached among Prince Boun Oum, Prince Souphanouvong, and himself, and that he had been selected to present his name to His Majesty the King as the prime minister of the new coalition government.

This was the breakthrough that most of those in Geneva had been hoping for, and they greeted the news with the belief that the work of the conference was near completion. But this was June, and the nations were going to have to prolong their Geneva meetings for nine months more.

What had not been settled at Hin Heup were the details of the new government, which faction should hold which cabinet positions. That may not have seemed a great obstacle, but it was. Then there were underlying reasons for one side or another to prefer to delay a final settlement.

The princes met again in December at Khang Khay on the kingdom's Plain of Jars, where the neutralists and the communists had camps. Boun Oum flew up from Vientiane, and this meeting endured for five hours before it disbanded with no agreement. They tried again at the end of December, when Prince Souvanna and Prince Souphanouvong flew down to Vientiane. This meeting was brief and unproductive.

A cartoon which appeared in the newspaper the *Providence Journal* during the Christmas holidays of 1961 depicted a temple scene in Laos with a written agreement for a coalition government lying in the center and the three princes indignantly walking their separate ways from it. The caption read: "We three princes of Orient are . . . adamant."

Months passed, and as an excuse for foot-dragging, Boun Oum demanded that his rightists control both the police and the army in the new government. This, he knew, would never be granted to him by either of the other factions or by the Geneva conference. It was a ploy to mark time and, while doing so, remain in control of Vientiane.

What Prince Boun Oum and General Phoumi Nosavan apparently failed to foresee was the growing impatience of the Pathet Lao. In May of 1962, Pathet Lao soldiers swept down on Phoumi's forces that were stationed at Houei Sai, a town near the Thai border. Phoumi's army repeated its previous track record and fled speedily, this time across the river to an alarmed Thailand. The Thai authorities feared that the communist soldiers might follow in pursuit. An emotional reaction to the Pathet Lao attack was also echoed in Washington. President Kennedy sent the Pacific fleet into nearby waters and quickly reached an accord with the Thai government to permit American soldiers to be based in Thailand. In this way, the Pathet Lao military action unwittingly engendered a most important strategic change in the region.

Faced by these actions and reactions, the Pathet Lao halted their advance.

In Washington, the rout at Houei Sai brought General Phoumi's military reputation to its nadir, even among those who had most ardently argued on his behalf.

Despite this, Phoumi and Prince Boun Oum continued their stalling tactics. It had been eight months since the Hin Heup meetings had agreed upon Prince Souvanna's leadership, and still the factions seemed no closer to actually forming a new government.

Souvanna Phouma was, as previously noted, quite different from most other national leaders. He had complete confidence in his ability to lead the country, but he was not seeking the position of ruler in order to fulfill ambitions or to fill a Swiss bank account. Therefore, if his leadership was not desired, or appreciated, he had no intention of forcing himself upon his people. And so in late May, Prince Souvanna announced that if the formation of a new government did not take place by June 15, he was going to leave the kingdom and retire in France.

The announcement created new waves of consternation in Geneva and elsewhere. The United States and other Western nations intensified their pressures on the Boun Oum–Phoumi Nosavan faction. Boun Oum protested but accepted another meeting.

Our three princes went back to the Plain of Jars and met once again, in the officers club at the Khang Khay airstrip. This time they took steps to constitute the new coalition government, and four days later, after daily sessions in the officers club, they announced the new cabinet.

Prince Souvanna Phouma was to be prime minister and minister of defense; Phoumi Nosavan, deputy prime minister and minister of finance; Prince Souphanouvong, deputy prime minister and economics minister. The ministers of the interior and of foreign affairs were to be neutralists, but the minister of information was to go to the Pathet Lao.

President Kennedy and Prime Minister Macmillan of Great Britain hailed the agreement, and none other than Soviet Premier Khrushchev praised the treaty and declared it could serve as a guide for other Western–Soviet bloc problems.

Did this mean the Geneva conference was now at an end? Not quite, but after a five-month recess, the representatives again gathered in the palace on the lake.

The nations, including the North Vietnamese, agreed that all foreign troops were to leave Laos except for a small French military training force, which would be allowed to remain. The North Vietnamese had had other soldiers spreading out over the little kingdom for years, and surely they never had any intention of abiding by the conference decision.

Another major issue that had to be determined was how and by whom the final resolutions of the conference would be observed and reported on. There was an unfortunate precedent: the 1954 Geneva conference on Indochina had established an International Control Commission to make on-the-spot inspections and to report on them. The ICC was composed of representatives of three countries: India, Canada, and Poland, with an Indian as chief commissioner. These commissions are still functioning, although very weakly. The original idea of such a body may have had much merit, and perhaps nothing better to replace it was suggested, but its bylaws had one overwhelming fault which rendered it almost hopeless: all decisions among the commissioners had to be unanimous.

How much would ever be accomplished if the decisions of our legislative and judicial bodies had to be unanimous? In the case of the ICC, which was primarily investigating communist incursions, to have a communist commissioner with the right of veto made it ludicrous. There had been many incidents of destruction and killings where investigation was called for, and when the Indian and Canadian commissioners had demanded action, the Pole had produced his veto. Here, after fifteen months of argument and discussion, a new International Control Commission was formed and given an assignment it could not realistically be expected to manage.

King Savang Vatthana went to Vientiane to preside on June 23, 1962, over the installation of the new neutralist government. The colorful ceremonies took place in the royal temple, where the *bonzes* sprinkled holy water over those who were about to assume their new positions.

On July 23, in the palace in Geneva, in a quiet ceremony, the conference came to its end. Representatives of the fourteen nations signed a document which concerned the ICC and its functions, prerogatives, and limitations. All of the representatives except for the Lao delegates signed a second document, which was a pledge to respect the neutrality of the little kingdom. That day's gathering in the palace lasted less than half an hour. The delegates were now free to return to their homes, and the little kingdom plunged once more into its perilous existence.

◆ ◆ ◆

In early 1961, before I could be sworn in as a foreign service officer, the Department of Education proposed that I go to Finland on a special four-month project. The idea was enticing, but I had my prior commitment with the Information Agency. However, the chief of personnel at the agency, a fine gentleman who had served in Helsinki, hearing of the situation, arranged for me to accept the grant and to be sworn into the agency on my return.

So off to Finland I went. The project necessitated traveling extensively throughout the country, even to Lapland. It was different from any place I had ever been—different but admirable. Finland, I learned, is a spacious land of birch trees and reindeer and scalding saunas from which one plunges into icy lakes.

On my return to Washington, I took my government oath and was informed that my first assignment was as branch public affairs officer in Savannakhet, the city south of Vientiane on the Mekong. Happy as I was at the thought of returning to Laos, I had reservations about residing in the stronghold of General Phoumi Nosavan.

By late summer of 1961, when the Geneva conference was still in its early stages, I was again in the little kingdom.

◆ ◆ ◆

No institution, I suppose, can escape politics. Certainly any college faculty has its intrigues—this group against that, this individual against that one. But within the academic community each member has, or supposedly has, a sense of devotion to studies and research.

I was quite unprepared for the outlandishness of some of the information agency officers I met within my first months in the service. I simply failed to understand them and could hardly believe that they were my new colleagues. I am speaking now of a few as opposed to most, but had I encountered these types while I was a grantee, I would have had second thoughts about leaving Hunter.

The first of these characters was in Washington—he was briefing me for my assignment to Savannakhet. I asked about transportation at that post and whether I should consider shipping my car overseas. The officer looked at me with grave suspicion and informed me that if I were planning to ship a car abroad at government expense in order to sell it at the post to make a fistful I had better forget it.

His remarks startled me. It suggested that the Foreign Service must be full of conniving scoundrels, that he himself may have been one, and that he was definitely judging me to be one. And this happened at a moment when I was looking forward to the service as nothing less than an inspiring calling.

When I arrived in Laos, I stayed in Vientiane for several days of further briefings. It was grand to be back in that city and to have fine reunions with old friends, Lao and Americans. But I was there in a new capacity and on the bottom of a chain of command: on top was the public affairs officer, who was the director of information services for the country, then his deputy, and finally, because I was to be at a field post, a field officer who was my supervisor. The PAO appeared to be a gentlemen and maybe a scholar, but he had other things on his mind and ignored me. The deputy was something else—a Mississippi man who even if he had worn a turtleneck could not have disguised how red his neck was. Even worse was his dear young friend, the field officer—he would swagger about wearing over his dirty khakis a gun belt, holster, and revolver. Evidently no one told him this was unlawful. For his part, he liked nothing better than to be mistaken for a Central Intelligence type, and tried to encourage the illusion. He often went to Savannakhet since that was the home of the Lao general he most admired. The field officer shared his lodgings with an attractive, youngish Chinese woman who was the madam for one of the most prominent brothels in Vientiane. She was far more likable than he was—at least I could have conversations with her.

There always is another viewpoint, and I realize how much the DPAO and the field officer must have disliked having the new branch officer turn out to be this New Yorker, this teacher of literature. Knowing that these two men constituted my major program support while in Savannakhet troubled me—and I was right to be so troubled.

◆ ◆ ◆

From China down to Cambodia, the Mekong courses through the little kingdom. In the wet season it becomes turbulent, gray, and ominous. Whatever happens to tumble in is carried downstream at a fast, relentless pace. Close to the Cambodian border, cascades make navigation treacherous for even the *pirogues*. By the end of the dry season, the great river appears to be no more than a wide, placid stream readily forded. Small islands are cultivated each winter only to disappear under the onrushing waters of springtime.

I have crossed the Mekong innumerable times, have taken boat rides both down to the frontier and up north above Luang Prabang to the Buddhist caves of Pak Ou, yet cannot easily explain my feelings about this river. It is not the visual delight and comforting presence that many rivers are. It is often majestic, but it maintains a mysterious air. It serves for many miles as a frontier—a frontier across which thousands have fled to safety, a frontier which today separates a communist state from a democratic state. I think from the first time I saw it, from the plane flying up from Bangkok, I sensed that the Mekong was somehow more than a river.

One aspect of it is fairly constant: on either side there are palm trees, rain trees, and thick jungle vegetation. The few cities of Laos are all situated on the banks of the river, necessitating in each instance that the green growth be cleared away to make room for an intrusive, mildly urban life.

Savannakhet is on a wide curve of the river, affording fine vistas of the Mekong both to the north and to the south. The sunsets over Thailand are often awesome in their brilliant colors.

But the city has little of historic interest. True, there is one fine temple of late Angkor period, but among the many other *wats*, while some are lovely, none compares to the exquisite *wats* of Luang Prabang or Vientiane.

In population, this is the third largest city of the kingdom. Its downtown area extends for perhaps a dozen blocks, and two-storied shop houses line the streets. The governor's offices are modest and provincial, the *lycée* is small and old, but the technical school is newer and larger. There are three movie houses but no cultural center, no formal cultural life. In the year before my arrival, two hotels had been built. Among the eating places, only one restaurant was worthy of that name, and it was not a good one.

Pakse, the city to the south of Savannakhet, and Thakhek, a town to the north of it, showed the French influence, and each had its certain charm, while Luang Prabang was uniquely and superbly Lao. Savannakhet lacked this sort of identification or affiliation. It was a modest, overgrown town, handsomely located on the Mekong, but with little else to recommend it.

Furthermore, its ambience was depressing because it had become so decidedly a military center. This was at the moment when American troops were at their greatest number in the kingdom. The people most in evidence were the soldiers, American and Lao, seeking recreation, and the whores who were providing them with an often boisterous sort of relaxation. The girls had come from everywhere in Southeast Asia. There were hundreds of them, and they could be found each evening in their flashy, clinging gowns entertaining the men in the many, many bars that had mushroomed in the city.

◆ ◆ ◆

Having had the good fortune to lead a life much to my liking, I feel it mean to complain about a brief part of it. Nevertheless, I shall mention some of the things that went wrong when I reached Savannakhet.

My lodgings consisted of a small room in a hotel where many American soldiers were billeted. The walls of the room did not extend to the ceiling, which meant that there was no privacy, and the electricity was so feeble, any effort to read in the evening resulted in eyestrain. Eating at the local restaurant soon made me quite physically sick.

The offices I inherited were a filthy mess, and what was supposed to have been the American library was a small pile of unassorted books, many of them of no interest to local readers. The young Lao in charge of the office, with whom the field officer was on friendly terms, was, I found out, stealing office funds and had to be dismissed.

I had been sent here to promulgate the American information program in the city and in the surrounding countryside, but I could not do that before I had dealt with this disarray. I faced a nasty challenge, especially since the support from Vientiane was so unsympathetic.

But I tried.

After six weeks, during which it had become increasingly difficult to eat or to sleep, I took off for a long weekend, went to Bangkok, and called on the old Danish doctor who was a fixture of that city. He examined me and listened to my tale of tribulations.

He asked, "How many tranquilizers are you taking each day?"

"I'm not taking any tranquilizers," I retorted as though insulted.

"Why not, you fool?" he commented in kind tones. He proceeded to write out a prescription for the pills to be picked up at the nearby British pharmacy.

Something else happened that weekend. A French teacher with whom I had been friendly when we both were on the faculty of the *Lycée de Vientiane* was now teaching in Bangkok and invited me to his home for dinner the first evening I was there. Also at dinner was a young French woman who was teaching her language at a Thai university. Her name was Anne-Louise. She was extremely sympathetic to my plight, and tender loving ears were exactly what I seemed to have been most in need of.

She and I spent the weekend together, and before I left, so comforted was I, that I asked Anne-Louise to come to Savannakhet and marry me, a rather drastic measure to overcome my gloom.

She did not say no, and I went back to Savannakhet in a far better frame of mind.

◆ ◆ ◆

Within another month, life in Savannakhet was altogether different. The United States Information Service moved to the best of the new downtown buildings. We had a truly attractive library and reading room on the ground floor with our offices upstairs. But to succeed in this type of public relations, all depends on personnel, and I was fortunate to gather together an excellent new staff.

The governor of the Thai province across the river invited me to a large party he was giving. While drinking beer and eating *satay*, I spoke with a young man who had just completed his university studies in India. His name was Pradit, and he was the son of a former deputy governor of the province. It was at once apparent that he was exceptionally bright and had a fine outgoing personality. He was planning to go to Bangkok to look for a position. I asked if working across the river could tempt him. He came over to our offices the next day, agreed to stay on, and became my first-rate assistant. It was enormously advantageous to have him help me cope with some of the situations that arose. Vientiane took notice of Pradit, and after I left he was given a position with the embassy, where he continued for another ten years.

For the library, we found a pretty and charming Lao girl with a *lycée* education. She did not know much about being a librarian, but she quickly learned. The *lycée* boys started to spend time at our reading room—her presence was largely responsible for this popularity.

My search for a house was initially frustrating. There was a large white concrete house that was vacant and, despite the need of much freshening, had the potential of being a good representational residence. The owner, a Lao army officer on General Phoumi's staff, said, when approached, that he had once rented it to some American army men and was not going to repeat that mistake. I tried persuasion—claimed that I was a diplomat, not a soldier—but he declined to make a commitment. He was, however, firm about the rent he demanded, and it would have been more appropriate for a fine East Side Manhattan townhouse. Alas, there was no choice.

I had to go to Vientiane for several days to attend a staff meeting. It is a rule, I presume, that the more insecure the director, the more frequent the long, useless meetings he inflicts upon his staff. When I got back to Savannakhet, Pradit was at the airport to meet me, and as we climbed onto the jeep said: "I think you had better look at the house."

"Why?" I inquired.

"You'll see," he replied.

I did see, and it was startling. I staggered to the door and peered inside—it was the same within. The owner, perhaps to make his house more valuable, perhaps to please me, or perhaps simply to please himself, had had the house painted in wide horizontal bands. The middle section was white, but up to the ceiling and down to the floor were heavy stripes of blue, green, yellow and red. The round concrete columns, an exterior and interior architectural element, were vivid pink. Never, anywhere in the world, have I seen a house painted in this fashion.

What to do? Yes, the owner had at last agreed to rent the house to me. Vientiane was not going to spend yet more money to redo it, nor could I ask the owner for a complete repaint, but it was certainly not my style to live in a concrete circus tent.

I groaned and groused, and every once in a while laughed uproariously.

The owner and I reached a very modest compromise. Some of the more vivid color would be muted, and one wide, purplish band near the floor would be whitened. But that was my Savannakhet house.

Fortuitously, I was able to bring down from Vientiane a Vietnamese couple. His name was Ky. He was deaf but more than compensated for his handicap by anticipating most requests, especially when serving at the table. He was also a diligent housecleaner. His wife, Mien, did the shopping and remarkably good French cooking. But she was an indomitable woman, and both Ky and I were wary of her. They also brought with them their four-year-old son, and although they kept him out of sight most of the time, his presence was a cheerful addition.

To be at last in my own house, with my books, some paintings and prints on the walls, and a stereo set, was a great satisfaction. There was a problem, albeit a minor one. In my limited supply of effects, I had sent only two phonograph albums: the *Brandenburg Concerti* and a new recording of *Don Giovanni* with London, Nilsson, and Price. And so I spent many an evening with nothing to do other than to sing along with Don or Ottavio or even Anna or Elvira.

A reporter from the *Bangkok Post* came into town to research a story on the Thai–Lao frontier. He called on me at my office, and I invited him home for dinner. Ky served drinks, Mien prepared a splendid meal, and we listened to Bach. The following week I read in the *Post* an article about a sybaritic expatriate American living in luxury in Savannakhet.

◆ ◆ ◆

What do you do if you happen to be branch public affair officer in Savannakhet? It is not easy to provide a rational response. You could sit in the office and do precious little, but that was not a possibility for me since I am plagued by a manic energy, inherited from my grandmother.

Consequently, I had to find activities, tasks to perform, people to meet, villages to visit. Because there was no consul in the city—no other official civilian American except for a USAID officer—as far as liaison between our embassy and the government and people of the province, I, to quote Alexander Haig, was in charge there.

Information means communications, and since we had no telephones, I had to reach USIS Vientiane twice a day by radio to let them know that no catastrophes had occurred and to learn whether they had any messages for me. They rarely did. The radio I had to use was located in the USAID officer's house, an attractive residence on the riverfront and less than a hundred yards from General Phoumi's home. The USAID officer was an elderly man, tall and lean with a dour disposition. He lived with a Vietnamese woman, younger than he, who saved him money by doubling as mistress and servant. In the year during which we were the only two American civilians in the city, and with my having to go to his house twice a day, he never invited me to partake of a meal with him, not even during those first months when I would have so welcomed such an invitation. Come to think of it, I don't believe he ever offered me a cup of coffee.

There was the radio, and then there was the milk run. This was the old DC-4 which flew down from Vientiane three times a week, delivering passengers and supplies before it continued on to Pakse and back to the capital. As BPAO, I was expected to be at the airport to meet the plane each time it flew in. It was also prudent for me to be there for one was never quite certain as to who or what might be aboard. Furthermore, it was a regular activity in a routine that needed activities.

The plane was often late, and I would engage in conversation with some of the Lao at the airport. One day an American officer came by and stared at me.

"What is it?" I demanded.

"Do you realize how you're sitting?"

Only then did I become aware that I was hunkering down as the Lao often did, and had probably been sitting on my heels for fifteen minutes or more without having paid any attention to my unlikely stance. That, I suppose, could be called going native.

Our Information Service in Vientiane printed fliers, magazines, comic books, and textbooks in Lao. These publications were then sent to the branch posts for distribution. In Vientiane we also had a film section where some documentaries were produced as well as many twenty-minute and half-hour films that told stories of Lao villagers who got into trouble by not taking sufficient precautions to protect themselves from the communists. It was my task to get as much of our material as we could manage out in the hinterlands. Accordingly, our two vehicles went out during the day distributing publications and in the evening showed films to the villagers.

For a sociologist, I believe that a Lao village should represent an almost ideal unit. The village chief was benevolent and respected. The members of the community grew rice and vegetables and raised pigs and poultry. The women wove cloth. The *wat* was both the religious and educational center, where the youngsters were taught by the *bonzes*.

The Lao village was a delightful place to visit. One often had to go through jungle trails to reach it, but there it would be—houses on poles, each with its veranda, a small temple, sometimes a small and primitive infirmary, and cultivated fields stretching out. The lovely women walked superbly in long, handsome skirts, their bosoms bare. The men sauntered about in their *pha khammas*, checked cotton cloths tied about their waists. The young children strutted about naked, while pigs and chickens and buffalo wandered much as they pleased.

When our jeep would come to the edge of the village, we would walk directly to the house of the chief. He, his legs covered with ornate Buddhist tattoos, would greet us and invite us to sit on the floor of his porch. A small cask of rice wine would be produced, and we would take turns sipping it through a community straw. If it were lunchtime, we would be invited to share their rice and whatever food was served with it. Bananas were always among the fruit.

Through an interpreter—Pradit if he were with me—I would inquire about the situation in the village. They sometimes had health concerns and sometimes needed assistance from USAID to dig wells for their dry season water supply. Occasionally they spoke of Pathet Lao movements in the area. Then I would present them with books and other publications.

An hour spent in a village with unfailingly pleasant people would always delight me. And I would think: How remarkable that I am here in this remote jungle village. Then sometimes there would be the added thought: But just what am I doing here?

The USIS officer in charge of the motion picture section in Vientiane, a talented, portly, jovial man who came to us from Denmark, once explained to me that the reason we had such tremendous turnouts whenever we went into a village to show our films was "because the villagers don't have another damned thing to do in the evenings."

◆ ◆ ◆

The American soldiers in Savannakhet were Green Berets, the group that John Wayne made into superheroes. They may not have fit that category, but they were by and large good men. They were here to help the little kingdom prepare to save itself from an enemy invasion, and most of them were serious in their mission and surprisingly sensitive to their assignment.

I am among those who believe there is nothing wrong in sending limited numbers of soldiers to train and strengthen a legitimate and friendly country that is being threatened. But let me add this caveat: In South Vietnam, from the time that President Johnson changed the basic concept and sent American troops not to train but to replace the local armies and to assume the fight against the North Vietnamese, I feared we were in deep trouble.

At the hotel in Savannakhet in which I initially stayed, the Green Berets had taken over the rooftop and converted it into an officers bar, the Bo Pen Yang, or "So What" club. The only decorations were two lines of colored lights suspended across the roof, but the site offered a grand view of the Mekong. Many an evening I drank beer, ate potato chips, and chatted away at the Bo Pen Yang.

When getting ready to leave New York for Savannakhet, some friends and I had attempted to gain admittance to the Peppermint Lounge, where Chubby Checkers and the twist had become a sudden and huge success, but we could not get into the establishment due to the long line at the door.

Shortly after I got to Savannakhet, I was on the roof with two captains who suggested we go to the Savannakhet Ratry, the leading local night spot. What a swinging joint it was, with a slick professional air. The decor was vivid red, the lighting dim and enticing, the round sunken dance floor large enough, the Filipino dance band pulsating, and the resident girls flamboyant in evening costumes. As we entered, the music was throbbing, and the American soldiers and girls on the dance floor were doing the twist. The twist: How had it gotten from the Peppermint Lounge to Savannakhet faster than I had? I stared at those dancers with their limber bodies swooping down close to the floor and then up again with tremendous vigor.

The band took a break, and when it resumed it played a *lam vong*. This I regretted. The gentle seductive rhythms of the Lao music that had never failed to entice me were here crudely syncopated, and the boys and girls moved their hands jerkily and waved their bottoms suggestively as they went around the circle. I was glad when this portion of the music ended and heard "Let's twist again." The Savannakhet Ratry was unexpected fun.

Our soldiers visited villages that were out of bounds for me unless I accompanied them, and so from time to time I went with them. One such trip was memorable. It was to two villages accessible only by river. We boarded a boat just large enough to transport a jeep and proceeded five miles downstream on a vast, sepia, choppy Mekong.

We passed some villages on the Thai side, but on the Lao side all we could see was an impenetrable growth. We beached the boat in a cove from which a trail barely wide enough for a vehicle led into the jungle. The soldiers got the jeep ashore while mosquitoes whirred and stung. Then we crowded our equipment and ourselves onto it and made our way inland.

Through the overhanging green came an occasional touch of sky—otherwise all was tree trunk and vegetation. Several times we were forced to halt while obstructing branches were removed. At one point we passed a sparkling, pale green pond with wide patches of coarse grass around it. The captain in charge of the expedition announced: "We'll stop here on the way back."

The trek took most of an hour until we reached the first village, simple and attractive. While the captain, his two aids, and I joined the chief on his veranda and sipped his rice wine, the two army medics—every army group that went to the villages had a pair of medics with them—took over the infirmary. A line of villagers formed at the entrance. Mothers carried infants, children stood impatiently, elders came with their complaints, and at the end of the line young men and women waited their turn for consultations. The medics gave time and distributed medicines to each person who wished to see them. The captain discussed security matters, and I gave those few textbooks I had been able to bring with me to a *bonze*.

We got back onto the jeep and continued on for another twenty minutes, when we stopped at a tiny clearing and walked down a path into the next village. The chief and other villagers were waiting for us, but in their midst was a tall, white-haired, Western woman who wore a Western-style blouse and skirt, eyeglasses, and a beneficent smile. She was a Swiss missionary who had lived here for more than five years. She invited us along with the chief and several others to her house, a structure just a bit larger than the others and resting on shorter poles.

The interior was neat and clean—she had not grown careless. As she served us tea and rice cakes, she spoke of the villagers with a devotion that was implicit, not flaunted. It seemed evident that the villagers cared deeply for her. She asked the medics to examine only two cases of illness, for she successfully tended the health problems of the community.

The woman mentioned that she had come to Laos in the hope of making some converts to Christianity, but that seemed less important to her now. Besides, she had grown comfortable with Buddhism. My trek into the jungle was an exotic adventure; her stay in the village was a humane and spiritual experience. I admired her greatly.

On the way back to the river, we stopped at that green pool and jumped in. Delicious, but the suspicion occurred there might be some nasty little creatures or organisms in that water. Fortunately, I suffered no ill effects.

We returned to the cove, loaded the jeep on the boat, and made our way upstream in waters that were calmer than they had been that morning. The soldiers had made this venture in order to check on security matters; they had looked around and done some questioning. But because they took medics with them, they were also performing a fine service for the villagers.

◆ ◆ ◆

I also took occasional trips to the villages with an American missionary. His name was Leslie.

Why anyone would wish to convert Buddhists befuddles me, but there were three sets of American missionaries in the city. The first were what might have been expected of certain nineteenth-century Protestants in Asia, a family group who lived in a typical Western house and held Sunday morning services in their home. They hoped to be able to build their own church but lacked sufficient converts to go to that expense. They were dull people who, I believe, assumed they were gaining points for the hereafter by living in this heathen land.

There were four Jehovah's Witnesses, two couples, young and, from my brief acquaintance with them, pleasant. They gave the impression that they, too, were not successful in their proselytizing.

Leslie was different. He was a handsome, vigorous man who had been a flyer during World War II. After the war, answering his inner need to devote himself to man and religion, he and his family came as missionaries to Laos. From his home in Savannakhet, he taught his neighbors how to keep themselves healthy and how to tend their vegetable gardens and farms. When he went out into the field, he was warmly greeted by the villagers, who regarded him as a friend there to help them. Furthermore, he spoke their language. I do not know whether Leslie tried to convert the Lao, but had he chosen to, he might have gained far more converts than the other missionaries.

◆ ◆ ◆

Until the Geneva conference came to its conclusion and its accords went into effect, it was General Phoumi Nosavan who controlled the Lao government. He spent most of his days in his new residence in Vientiane, or on travels abroad, but from time to time we in his hometown of Savannakhet had the dubious honor of his presence.

Once he came for what might best be described as a pep rally. The newest and largest cinema house was filled to capacity with townspeople and soldiers. But these were troubled moments for the extreme rightists of Laos, and this assembly of disciples reflected the malaise.

Two generals addressed the audience, and then Phoumi spoke to them. He was not a good orator, but his tone conveyed the conviction and assurance of one who had determinedly fought his way to power. The crowd applauded, but he failed to rouse them to anything like the ovation Captain Kong Le had received after having overthrown a previous Phoumi Nosavan government.

The rally lasted no more than two hours, and then the crowd dispersed quietly, calmly. I came across my old friend Ambassador Nouphat as he was leaving the theater, and we exchanged cordialities and generalities. He did not wish to discuss the significance of this gathering—no one seemed to want to do that.

A few weeks later I received an invitation for the wedding reception of Phoumi's niece. It was to be held at his local residence.

On that afternoon, many tables and chairs were arranged on the wide lawn on the riverbank. Each guest was assigned to the section that befitted his stature, and, therefore, most were on the green. Inside the house, in the salon and dining room, were certain older, distinguished relatives and representatives from the palace in Luang Prabang, or from Prince Boun Oum's Champassak, or from across the river in Thailand. Foreign guests, such as myself, were received on the veranda.

The general went from the house to the porch and back inside. He seemed to ignore those on the lawn. He spoke with a few American military officers and then addressed me: "Are you enjoying Savannakhet?"

"Yes," in two syllables, an effort in discretion (to mark my reluctance in replying).

"As much as you enjoyed living in Vientiane?"

Surprised, I said something about liking Vientiane, but avoided making the comparison he was demanding. Phoumi turned and gave his attention to another of his guests.

How did he know that I had at one time lived in Vientiane? I could not recall having mentioned that in any of our previous brief conversations. Had he been checking on me? Had I made some unfavorable remark about him or his government that had been reported back to him? Didn't he realize that my being branch public affairs officer in Savannakhet meant that I was the low man on the official American totem pole? Or was I in such a strange environment that I was inflating the significance of an innocent remark? Years later I was to learn at least in part the answer to my musings about Phoumi suspicions.

◆ ◆ ◆

Another duty in the domain of a BPAO was one for which I was hardly qualified: to escort American journalists to where the fighting was taking place. But then, was anyone qualified for this task?

Three correspondents arrived at my house. They were fed and bedded, and in the morning the four of us took off in a jeep-wagon north to Thakhek, a town on the Mekong. The French had been there, and the French had left their handsome mark upon it. The streets were wide and lined with trees. The colonial architecture that remained had a poignant charm, especially the local inn, The Bungalow. Unfortunately, while this long, low structure on the river's edge was remarkably attractive, it was in the furthest state of decay of any lodging in which I have ever tried to sleep. At night, it was not a precaution but a necessity to place all of one's belongings on the bed with the mosquito netting tucked in under the bumpy mattress and hope that the large rats which romped about were not going to tear their way through the netting. After my initial visit to Thakhek, I had tried to avoid spending nights there, but with the journalists on this trip, the ordeal could not be escaped.

The next day we visited the local army headquarters and eventually continued on to a village close to Pathet Lao territory. We slept that night on bedrolls on the porch of the village chief's house, an arrangement infinitely preferable to lodging at the inn at Thakhek.

From the village, an American lieutenant arranged for us to go in the jeep of a young Lao soldier to the very area where Phoumi's soldiers and the Pathet Lao had been exchanging gunfire. The lieutenant wished us luck as we went off by ourselves—not entirely unescorted, for I was officially designated as the escort.

The jeep came to a halt. We descended and walked about on the side of a hill. There was no habitation, no sign of life. A small stream was beneath us, and on the other side was another hill covered by thick vegetation with some clearings. The soldier artlessly informed us that that was where the enemy was.

Then to my great surprise, he told us he was leaving us for a while—had some urgent matter to tend to. Before I could discuss or argue his decision, he was in his jeep and away.

The journalists quite naturally asked me what they were to do now. I had no logical answer. We strolled a bit, but not far, not wishing to distance ourselves from this quite undistinguished spot. It was hot, and eventually we sat in the shade of a rain tree.

The ugly sound of shooting destroyed the quiet. More shots. They were loud and seemed to come from an uncomfortably close distance.

"Gentlemen," I said in a feeble attempt at humor, "here we are, just as we wished to be, right at the scene of action."

A long period of silence ensued. Some attempts on my part to engage the group in conversation, to talk about politics or the Geneva conference or anything, failed dismally.

Time dragged on torturously. Never has it loitered so. I was developing a cramp in my wrist from constantly turning it to look at my watch. It was one hour since the driver had left us.

On the other side of the stream, two men came out of the woods to cross a clearing. They were not dressed as villagers in *pha khammas,* nor were they in uniform. They wore trousers and shirts, and they carried rifles. They saw us, stopped, and stared at us. Their expressions, as best we could make out, were not threatening, but neither were they friendly. The four of us moved as little as possible during this interlude. After what seemed many minutes, the two men continued on their way and back into the thicket.

"Stieglitz, what have you gotten us into?" one of the newsmen grumbled. His question echoed precisely my thought.

Two hours.

We were trapped. If the Pathet Lao wanted to capture four Americans, there we were—easy pickings. And why were we there, unarmed, on their territory?

None of us expressed our feelings. I had to maintain some pretense that this was not an alarming situation. Any frantic sentiments I harbored had to remain deep inside.

More than two and a half hours after he had deposited us there, the driver returned. He explained that he had taken two wounded soldiers to a village where they could be treated. We were supposed to be grateful that he had not forgotten us entirely.

Back in my house in Savannakhet that evening, we consumed a lot of whiskey. We deserved it.

◆ ◆ ◆

Anne-Louise came to Savannakhet. She had not, fortunately, resigned her teaching position with the intention of remaining with me but had made the excursion during a school vacation.

Happy to see and to be with each other, we were nevertheless well aware of how fragmentary was our understanding of each other. But in Savannakhet, with so few outside distractions, we could advance at supersonic speed from acquaintanceship to that stage of clinical knowledge which the psychiatrist is apt to attain only after his patient has been on his couch for many months.

Ky served us Mien's meals three times a day, and we listened to some records for the phonograph Anne-Louise had brought with her. We were invited out once, and she pretended to find the party amusing, although it was hardly in her conventional milieu: the men were American military officers, and the woman were girls from the bars and night club.

One afternoon we went by jeep to Seno, a forty-five-minute drive which necessitated our passing through a series of barrier-gates. At each of them armed guards checked us out before allowing us to proceed. She accepted this intimation of danger in stride.

I used to go to Seno occasionally because the French *économat*, or commissary, was there. While we Americans were often embarrassingly difficult about permitting anyone without all the credentials to purchase anything in our commissary, the French could not have been more generous in giving me the right to buy whatever was available in theirs. Since my only way of getting provisions from Vientiane was to request them via that radiophone and then accept what was sent whenever it happened to get to me, I was especially grateful to be able to shop in Seno. Furthermore, sometimes available at the *économat* would be such delicacies as *gigot* (frozen, to be sure), *flageolets* (tinned, but delicious), and *foie gras*.

Anne-Louise and I lunched at *the* restaurant of Seno. Its appearance was drab, but the dozen tables were set with white linen and wineglasses, and the aromas that wafted out of the kitchen were irresistible. The patron was courteous and friendly. His unusal customers were French pilots and army officers, and he seemed delighted to have as a guest a young Frenchwomen he had not previously seen. He hovered over us, asking Anne-Louise where she was from and what she was doing in remote Seno. We ate a delicious *pâté de campagne* and *côtes de veau* accompanied by a fine Mersault. It was an excellent meal and a pleasant day.

But the relationship between Anne-Louise and me was definitely uneasy. This was not because of our religious difference, although she was raised a devout Catholic and I am Jewish. What did separate us was that in her concept of religion, suffering was a predominant element of life.

In our day and age, when we contemplate the future, only a fool can be an optimist. However, passive acceptance runs counter to my fiber. I know we all must suffer, we all must face ultimate defeat, but the refusal to accept the inevitable is, for me, the stuff of life.

The more I peered into her eyes, the sadder they revealed

themselves to be. The more she looked at me, the more she surely realized the chasm between us.

By the time she left Savannakhet, a budding relationship was rapidly fading.

◆ ◆ ◆

The government circle in Vientiane—that area touching on the grounds of the National Assembly, the *lycée*, and other government buildings, that quiet circle in which I had seen buffalo roam and once wild horses run—was being converted into the site of a vast monument. Although its basic form was that of a huge arch in the French style, it was so elaborately overdecorated as to be silly. Phoumi Nosavan was responsible for this—a monument to immortalize him. He called it an *arc de triomphe* (the Lao promptly dubbed it Phoumi's Folly and unofficially renamed Avenue Lan Xang, that wide boulevard that led from the river to the arch, Phoumistrasse).

An *arc de triomphe de mauvais goût* it was, but through the years the arch has seemed to take on a sort of Disneylandish charm.

In August 1962, a grand parade was hastily organized to celebrate the signing of the Geneva accords and the installation in Vientiane of the neutralist tripartite government. The parade was scheduled to proceed up the avenue to the monument.

This was to be a unique moment in the little kingdom's history: soldiers representing General Phoumi's army, Kong Le's valiant forces, and the Pathet Lao were going to participate in a peaceful manifestation. Neutralist and communist troops were flown in from the north for this event.

Although Phoumi was no longer head of government, he had the manpower to remain more or less in charge of the city. Feeling something akin to embarrassment upon seeing all those potholes that punctuated the avenue, Phoumi ordered that this condition be remedied immediately. Accordingly, the night before the parade there was much activity on the thoroughfare. Trucks poured asphalt, and rollers smoothed it down.

Kong Le's troops came down from the Plain of Jars in the morning, and their uniforms were pathetic. A generous American officer decided to do something for them and requisitioned as many pair of paratrooper boots as he could. These were distributed to the soldiers. That the boot in almost all cases were many sizes too large for their small feet hardly mattered. The boots were to serve the day.

The sun shone fiercely. Even by Vientiane standards it was excessively hot. By the time the parade began, Avenue Lan Xang was a pool of thick, hot tar.

The soldiers marched bravely, trying to keep time to the drummer's beat. But walking on that asphalt was a formidable task. Their feet were sinking in and had to be awkwardly pulled out.

For Kong Le's men, the parade became an especially challenging obstacle course. One soldier's American boots sank in intractably, and the spectators saw him bend down quickly to unlace them. He continued on, poor fellow, in bare feet, which alleviated not at all the problem of marching on tar. Then the crowd noticed another pair of boots abandoned in the middle of the avenue, and another. Soon the pavement was decorated by many empty boots.

Eventually, most of those participating reached the arch and beyond it, congratulating themselves on having completed the course.

The parade formed a major part of the celebration, and one wag quipped that the new government had been launched in asphalt. Would that it had been!

A few days later, on August 20, a meeting of the new cabinet was held at the prime minister's villa, a large, white stucco house surrounded by palms and hibiscus and located close to the king's Vientiane palace. Although Prince Souvanna Phouma had his personal office in his house, it was too small to accommodate the cabinet. They therefore met in his long, tall-columned dining room, where the ceiling fans provided a continuous soft whir.

The date was significant because two days later, on the twenty-second of the month, the government was to give to the International Control Commission certain details concerning the departure of the foreign troops. And then, within forty-five days, by midnight on October 7, all troops, with the exception of a small French military training unit, were to have left the country. This timetable had been established as a primary part of the Geneva accords.

As they sat about the dining room table, the cabinet agreed that

the American soldiers would depart on October 7 from both
Vientiane and Savannakhet. The four hundred Filipino military
technicians would have gone before then. As for the thousands—
perhaps ten thousand—of North Vietnamese soldiers, when
would they be leaving, and from where? All attention focused on
Prince Souphanouvong, who was, in a very real sense, the spokesman for the North Vietnamese. He and Hanoi had always insisted
that there were no incursive Vietnamese troops in Laos. How
could he now admit that they would be leaving? And since the
North Vietnamese were dispersed throughout the country, sometimes in areas that were almost inaccessible, and since any attempt
to investigate their presence was vetoed by a Polish commissioner,
Hanoi's outrageous denials would be difficult to prove.

The atmosphere in the room grew tense. Souphanouvong
maintained to a good measure his unperturbable manner, but
those who knew him well could detect his discomfort. Phoumi
Nosavan fumed and threatened. Souvanna tried his superb diplomacy to induce an admission from his half-brother. Quinim
Polsena, the minister of foreign affairs, whose neutrality was
suspect because of his sympathetic attitude toward the Pathet Lao,
said little, even though he knew that a failure to give the
commission the required information would endanger the fif-
teen-month work of the fourteen nations. The meeting ended
acrimoniously.

Prince Souvanna asked Prince Souphanouvong to remain
when the others left. The two spoke, sipped wine, and dined. The
princes, politically antithetical, maintained strong family ties. A
close relative of theirs once remarked that it was unfortunate that
Souvanna, whose perceptions were generally so acute, failed to
recognize the Macbeth-like qualities of the Souphanouvongs.

That evening, Souphanouvong informed Quinim Polsena and
later the press that yes, there were some North Vietnamese and
Soviet advisers in the kingdom, approximately fifty, and they, too,
would leave on October 7. Their departure point would be the
Plain of Jars.

October 7 happened coincidentally to be the prime minister's
birthday, his sixty-first, and at a reception in his honor, he stated:
"We should despite everything rejoice without reserve that one of
the most important clauses of the Geneva accords, which refers to

the departure of foreign troops from Laos, is being observed according to the wishes of the signatory nations." In Washington, Averell Harriman also expressed some optimism based on his belief that the Soviets wanted to have the Geneva agreements carried out. But neither Souvanna nor Harriman could be certain that during that particular period the Soviets were able to control the actions of the North Vietnamese or the Pathet Lao.

On that day, three control commissioners were on the Plain of Jars to check out the fifty communist soldiers as they left. Most of the commissioners were in Vientiane to observe most of the American soldiers take their departure. And we had our very own ceremony at the airport of Savannakhet.

Two military transport planes waited as three commissioners, an Indian, a Canadian, and a Pole, took their places on the tarmac. The governor, two generals, and other Lao military and civilian officials plus onlookers crowded the scene.

The American soldiers arrived. Their uniforms were sharply pressed, their brass buckles brightly polished, and their postures as erect as West Pointers on parade. They marched smartly in single file past the commissioners, saluting as they did, and continued onto the planes. The commissioners counted each of them. As soon as the last soldier was aboard, the planes roared down the field and into the air, leaving Savannakhet a very changed city.

Later, walking home from my office, I passed the hotel where our soldiers had been billeted. It was lifeless. I had dinner, then stepped out of the house to walk about town.

The bars were all open. As usual, music blared forth from each, and girls in flashy, provocative dresses stood or sat, looking to the street in anticipation. But the customers were missing. I must have felt somehow guilty, for I made a foolish little effort: I would enter a bar, exchange hearty greetings, order and pay for a drink or two, chat a bit, and then go on to the next bar. That attempt to dispel the gloom was ridiculous. The girls knew their Lao experience had come to an end, but the end had arrived so abruptly, they had not yet reconciled themselves to it. They would spend another evening or two at the bars, listening for rumors of where more American soldiers could be found. Then they would decide where next to try their fortunes, and how to get there.

Within days, the hopes in Vientiane for the kingdom's post–

October 7 status were greatly dampened, if not extinguished. From Hanoi and from Beijing came loud claims that the Americans had not left, that American soldiers remained in the kingdom in disguise. No one bothered to ask: disguised as what? Almost everyone seemed to understand why these claims were being made: since the Americans had complied with the Geneva accords and Hanoi had not, promulgating false charges was one way to confuse the issue.

◆ ◆ ◆

General Boun Pone was the commander of the southern armies of the little kingdom. He was a native of Champassak, and his pretty wife was a niece of Prince Boun Oum. He was at a comparatively young age the epitome of the Champassak establishment figure.

He was short and stocky but had an air of elegance. His khaki uniforms looked as though they had been tailored for him on Saville Row. In a country were many were gracious, he was particularly so.

One of my duties was to maintain relations with the Lao military leaders in the area, and I often had reason to call on him at his army headquarters. He would always find time to chat. He was intelligent and sensitive, and more relaxed than most military leaders I have known. He had been educated abroad and had a worldly knowledge of foreign affairs. Conversations with him convinced me that he was far more concerned with keeping the kingdom out of communist clutches than with advancing the rightists' ambitions. If I regretted that he was one of Phoumi Nosavan's top generals, I was pleased that such a man occupied that position.

We became friends, and when I entertained at home, he was often among my guests. The other highest-ranking officials in Savannakhet were the governor of the province and the general of the regional army. My relations with both of them were good, but hardly in the friendship category.

A change vastly for the better occurred in Vientiane when the public affairs officer and his deputy were replaced. The two new arrivals promptly decided that I should be in Vientiane for the remainder of my assignment in Laos, and I was happy at the prospect. The move was scheduled for the beginning of November, but this was still mid-October, the American soldiers had left the city, and it was time for the annual water festival, a joyous Lao event with religious connotations.

A permanent pavilion, a long open structure without walls but with columns and a roof, stood directly on the edge of the riverbank in the center of Savannakhet. This pavilion served as the focal point of the festival. On the evening preceding the holiday, the generals entertained there. Temporary tents, actually colored parachutes held up by bamboo poles, extended from the pavilion. We, the guests, sipped rice wine, beer, or whiskey, and watched the remarkable spectacle on the river. Hundreds of tiny rafts made of bamboo or banana wood, each covered with fancy and often original decorations and each illuminated ingeniously by diminutive oil lamps, were launched and floated downstream. The great Mekong was transformed into an enchanting, sparkling sea, and delectable Lao music added to the magic of the scene.

As the last of those lights on the water drifted away, we were summoned to huge buffet tables under the tents. We were eating and talking and the musicians were performing when, with an incredible suddenness, a wild rain and wind storm swooped down upon us. Many of us dashed for shelter under the open pavilion, and in moments the colorful tents had been torn from their poles and had fallen into the instantly created mud. We huddled together for half an hour, by the end of which we were completely drenched, our clothes clinging to us as though we had just emerged from the river. But true to the Lao character, there was much laughter and no grumbling. No one cursed the elements or swore at his neighbor for stepping on him. Quite abruptly, the storm stopped and allowed us to go to our homes and peel off our clothing.

We returned the next afternoon for the boat races. The pavilion, gaily redecorated, was now the grand reviewing stand. Reserved seats were arranged under its roof, the first row composed of comfortable armchairs for the two generals, the governor, and a few others. Boun Pone came to where I was standing and, to my surprise, led me to one of those very important chairs.

The Lao are sometimes accused of being leisurely paced, even lazy, but when it is time for holiday festivities, these are a people of enormous energy and creativity. The boats for the races were the traditional *pirogues*, long canoes that carry merchandise up and down the river. For this occasion, each town or trade group had a boat to represent it, and the craft were brightly painted and adorned with a profusion of flags. Each was manned by a crew of twenty, and most of the crewmen were also rompishly attired. Some with minimal resources wore only their *pha khammas*, but most were bedecked in vividly colored shirts and pants with matching headscarves or festooned straw hats.

The races pitted two boats in each contest, and the winners would compete against each other. It was astonishing to see how skillful they were: these men with no real training and using the crudest of oars cut through the water with the speed and precision of a scientifically coached college crew. Between races, another aspect of Lao popular culture was flaunted, a love of rabelaisian humor. Clowns entertained, and many of them sported large, false phalluses, which they flashed and joked about. Others performed as zany transvestites. The spectators thoroughly enjoyed this humor—in this context, it was not offensive.

The races were over, and the winners came forward to receive their prizes. During this ceremony, again totally unexpectedly, I was called upon to bestow one of the awards. That day I felt so comfortably a part of the community, I almost started to regret my forthcoming departure from the city.

A few days later, Boun Pone came by my office. He and his wife were going to Champassak for the weekend and wanted me to join them. What a special invitation that was!

The three of us flew from Savannakhet to Pakse in the general's own small aircraft. A car waited there to take us down along the river on a narrow and sometimes bumpy but adequate road. Within an hour we reached a ferry, a raft-type craft capable of carrying two vehicles at a time. As we crossed the water, I had my first view of Champassak.

Four, large, white-frame houses faced the river, and the effect was precisely like that of a New England summer resort. When I looked further there were, to be sure, elsewhere in the village, typical Lao houses, but those four dominated the scene. They sat on a wide, calm stretch that made the Mekong seem a grand lake.

These houses belonged to the princes of Champassak. I was given a room in one, a pleasant room overlooking the river and, to my mind, again with the flavor of a northern American resort.

Before dinner, Boun Pone gathered some fifteen of us on the wide veranda of one of the houses for drinks. A servant offered helpings of a certain Lao dish which I recognized as raw pork pâté. There was, I feel certain, nothing dangerous about this food, but my hygienic American background refused to allow me to taste it. Casually, I said no to the pâté, but not inconspicuously enough for the eye of my host. Soon the servant returned with a plate of fried eggs and offered them to me. I started to refuse, but he insisted, and not wishing to create any embarrassment, I took the eggs. Boun Pone came by smiling and mentioned that he knew I would not eat the raw pork and this was a substitute dish. I had always believed that he was a man of sensitivity. This little incident confirmed that premise.

We had dinner at Prince Boun Oum's house and afterward went to a public garden next to the river, where an evening entertainment was in progress. There was the dance platform, the musicians, and the *lam vong*. We sat at tables or danced. The moon was huge, and its reflection shimmered in the Mekong. The setting was lovely, the company delightful, the music captivating.

The next morning, several of us went in jeeps farther south along the river on a dirt road to the ruins of the ancient temple, Wat Phu, a structure of the Khmer period. On the side of a hill overlooking a small lake are two oblong halls built of the thick dark stone with heavily framed windows that characterize the great temples of Angkor. But Wat Phu has its own little miracle of beauty. Between the halls rises a flight of stone stairs which leads to an intimate temple built of the same stone but of the most delicate proportions. You climb the stairs and enter this remnant of a personal temple, you look down across the countryside to the lake and the river valley beyond, you are transported in time back some ten centuries. It is thrilling to find another instance where man and nature have sublimely complemented each other.

We spent some time wandering about the site. Below the halls, my foot struck an object protruding slightly from the ground. Curious, I dug with my hands until I was able to pick up the fair-sized stone object. It was a Khmer torso, one of those prized treasures such as may be found in the great art museums. I held it in my arms and experienced simultaneously joy and dismay. No one was close to me at that moment, but obviously I could not take this statue with me, not even with the intention of presenting it to a museum. It wasn't mine, but it did not belong to anyone except to its surroundings, and there it had been ignored for years or, more likely, centuries. If I were to call it to the attention of Boun Pone or one of the other officials with whom I was making the trip, what would he do with it? Keep it in his own possession? That would be as likely as leaving it in the ground. But I wanted it left at Wat Phu. I wanted it to be visible to those few who came to this temple. But there was no museum here, no place to leave it. I returned it to its hole in the ground and hoped that on some future date, this magnificent sculpture might resume its place in that gem of a temple.

We returned to Champassak for one more night before flying back to Savannakhet. A few days later, I left that city for Vientiane.

Now let us for a moment advance through the years. In 1967, I was once more in Laos and about to be married to the daughter of a northern Lao prince. For several reasons, my bride-to-be and I had made no announcement of our plans, but the rumor mills were grinding away. One evening at a large reception, Boun Pone and I saw each other for the first time in years. There was a warm grasp of hands and shoulders, and then, almost at once, he said: "My friend, I want you to know that I am very happy for you, even though you are marrying into the *other* family."

In 1975, when the North Vietnamese took over the little kingdom, the Lao understandably reacted in various ways. Boun Pone made no effort to flee or to excuse his having been the head of the Southern Armies. He was among the many sent up north to a so-called reeducation camp. And he was among those who never returned from the camp, and never will return. Rest, general. Peace!

◆ ◆ ◆

On my first day as information officer in Vientiane, in November 1962, the administration man drove me in his jeep to see the house that would be mine. We went along the river, past the scarlet flame trees, and continued on the road as it veered inland south toward Thadeua and the ferry. But before we left the city limits, we turned to the right on a lane that ran some hundred yards to the Mekong. Halfway down this lane, we took a driveway to an old wooden one-story house surrounded by frangipani, hibiscus, and bougainvillaea, a bright potpourri of a garden.

The house itself had a spacious odd-shaped living room with a dining area and only one bedroom. This limited it for representational purposes, but the salon and the garden were large. The servants' quarters behind were ample.

I was ready to move in at once, but my good housekeepers, Ky and Mien, who came up from Savannakhet with me, informed me that I would have to stay elsewhere for several days until they had scrubbed the house and their quarters sufficiently to meet their standards. At last I was allowed to move in, and in style. The first evening, Ky served me my before-dinner drink and then the delicious repast that Mien had prepared.

In the morning I rose very early—as is my bad habit—and stepped outside as seven *bonzes* made their way past the house on their way toward the river. They formed a procession, single file, saffron-robed, feet bare or sandaled, with two of the older ones carrying open black umbrellas to shade them. Each monk held in his arms a large silver bowl. From the few other houses on the lane, women emerged with baskets of offerings, then knelt and placed food in their silver bowls as the holy men went by. This procession of the *bonzes* and the presentation of the food by the faithful is a daily ritual. The monks eat only in the morning and only that provided in this fashion. Furthermore, the *bonzes* do not thank those who give: rather it is the givers who thank them for this opportunity to gain merits.

Later I walked down the lane and realized that my property was adjacent to the grounds of Wat Phyawat. All of the space from my house to the river belonged to the temple. The principal building, the place of worship, was not particularly impressive, and the dwellings of the *bonzes* that radiated from it were small and simple. But in the midst of the green lawn and dominating the scene sat a splendid stone Buddha, perhaps twenty-five feet in height. He was impassive and sublime with a trace of a smile on his heavy lips. His legs were crossed in front of him, and the long fingers of one hand rested on one foot, while the other hand fell across a knee. A palm tree had pushed up behind him, wreathing his face in green foliage.

This Buddha had originally been within a large wooden temple, but the building had collapsed, possibly eroded by termites. Years after I inhabited the lane, another temple was built to house him, suggesting his importance to the worshipers. While I lived there, as an immediate neighbor and frequent visitor, I came to look upon this solemn yet somewhat amused god as my Buddha.

Each *wat* had its annual *boon*, or fair, which served as both a religious celebration and as a fund-raising event. This fact of temple life became vividly evident all too soon after I moved in when the lane was abruptly transformed into a superhighway of sorts. Pedestrians, bicycles, pedicabs, autos, and trucks paraded by on their way to prepare for the *boon* at Wat Phyawat. Those quiet grounds were brusquely converted into a huge bazaar.

Despite having observed the frenetic preparations, I was still unprepared for the opening evening, when masses of people converged on the lane, and the roar of the sound systems was ear-splitting. Colored lights criss-crossed the grounds, and hawkers' cries competed with the loudspeakers that conveyed the voices of performing musicians or that accompanied the film projections. Several platforms for dancers had been erected. The activities began in late afternoon and continued vigorously and clamorously until three in the morning.

To sleep the first night I had to put cotton in my ears. I had to do the same on the second and third nights. On the fourth evening I attended a dinner party, and present there were good friends who also lived on the lane, the French artist Jean-Pierre Geoffroy Dechaume and his wife, Yvonne. We naturally discussed our sleeping problems and decided how best to survive. We gathered some others from the dinner and proceeded to the fair. There, eventually, we settled in a clearing close to the river where a scattering of tables and chairs surrounded a dance floor. The music was playing. Two by two we stepped onto the platform and became part of the *lam vong* circle: hands seductively inviting, then rejecting. Around and around—we danced around—hands and music, music and hands. We were Lao.

Hours later as I started back to my house, I paused in front of my Buddha. Despite the noise and frenzy, he remained all wisdom and tranquility.

❀ ❀ ❀

In their attempt to rule the little kingdom with a tripartite government, the neutralists faced innumerable, almost insuperable, problems. The rightists and the communists ran a gamut of attitudes from uncooperative to hostile, and within the neutralist party itself, a conflict erupted.

General Kong Le, for the little captain had been elevated to this lofty rank, had his troops on the Plain of Jars. General Phoumi Nosavan had his army ensconced in Vientiane and was determined to keep the neutralist army at a distance. But in order to provision the neutralists, planes carrying their needs had to be flown up to the Plain of Jars. Since the Lao air force was still under Phoumi's direction, it could not be entrusted with this duty, and American military transport planes were pressed into service.

The use of American military planes in Laos was in violation of the Geneva accords, and a violation is a violation is a violation. Nevertheless, the United States was acting in this matter at the request of Souvanna Phouma's government.

Furthermore, extenuating conditions were noted: one so frivolous as the rice drop was not a military use of the plane; one as tit-for-tat as Hanoi had never complied with the accords, had never withdrawn its troops; and one as ominous as Washington and Hanoi were making preparation for war in South Vietnam. All true, and yet a violation is . . .

Soon after I moved back to Vientiane, an American plane bringing rice to Kong Le's troops was shot down. The man responsible for the destruction of the plane and the consequent killing of its occupants was Colonel Deuane, a neutralist army officer. Deuane had become increasingly allied to the communists, and following the shooting he and several of his men hurriedly defected to the Pathet Lao.

Colonel Ketsana Vongsanovah was chief of staff of the neutralist army on the Plain of Jars. A young man, only thirty, he was an ardent supporter of the political philosophy of Prince Souvanna Phouma and of General Kong Le, his immediate superior. Ketsana deplored Deuane's nefarious deed and went to the Pathet Lao camp to demand that Deuane be returned to the neutralists for disciplinary measures. The Pathet Lao countered that Deuane and his men had asked for and received sanctuary with them. Ketsana's request was angrily denied.

In December an attempt was made on Ketsana's life, but it failed. Two months later, Ketsana was in the village of Ponsavan on the Plain of Jars when he was stalked and killed by a group of Pathet Lao assassins.

This murder begot murder.

Quinim Polsena had been a leading member of the neutralist delegation to the Geneva conference. He had been born in Laos of a Lao mother and a Chinese father who was among the merchants in Vientiane. While in his teens, Quinim became a ward of the Souvanna Phouma household, not an unusual occurrence in the kingdom, where prominent families for various reasons might accept talented young persons as protégés. It was then natural that he became a civil servant and eventually, with Prince Souvanna's assistance, governor of the northern province of Samneua.

Quinin was an ambitious man, readily flattered and easily offended. As he rose to prominence, he was invited to join several overseas missions. While in the United States, he felt he was slighted by the Americans, but his ego was bolstered by the fuss the Soviets made about him in the USSR. Apparently this slight and that praise deeply influenced him. He entered into politics, was elected to the National Assembly, and then formed his own splinter party with a proleftist cast. This led to his defeat for the Assembly in 1960 and separated him further from the rightists, who were the overwhelming victors in the spurious election.

He took up the merchant's life and ran a gunsmith shop in Vientiane. When Kong Le led his *coup d'état* against Phoumi, Quinim hurried to the young captain's side and offered him political advice. When Phoumi's forces attacked in the infamous Battle of Vientiane, it was Quinim who hastened to bring in the Pathet Lao on the side of the neutralists. He joined Kong Le in defeat on the Plain of Jars.

Some believe that while negotiations were underway in Geneva, the Pathet Lao and their North Vietnamese mentors were more inclined to accept Souvanna's proposed cabinet because Quinim was to be named foreign minister.

Early in 1963, His Majesty King Savang Vatthana and Prince Souvanna Phouma went abroad to make courtesy calls on several of the nations which had taken part in the Geneva conference, including the United States, the Soviet Union, and China. Quinim, as minister of foreign affairs, accompanied them.

On the first day of April, the king held a reception in his Vientiane palace. The occasion was the end of the journeys and the launching of a new peace effort among the three Lao factions. The weather was pleasant that evening as several hundred guests in formal attire strolled about the palace, the riverside pavilion, and the carefully tended grounds. However, those who attended noticed an absence of the customary Lao joviality.

William Hamilton, the American political officer at the embassy, happened to be standing near the entrance hall when Quinim and his wife prepared to leave. Before their departure, Hamilton spoke to the minister briefly and found him to be quite his usual self, that is, abrasive but otherwise at ease.

Quinim and his wife were driven to their residence, which was not far from the palace. As they walked up the few steps to the door of their house, a young soldier, a bodyguard, nineteen years old, raised his gun and shot and killed Quinim. His wife was wounded by stray bullets that hit her legs.

The soldier was a Corporal Kong, a neutralist. Little else is known. In Southeast Asia, as in much of the non-Western world, a public event is not always open to public scrutiny. In the case of Corporal Kong, a curtain fell quickly.

But there are questions. Was this young man aware of the statement made several days before by General Kong Le in his headquarters at Khang Khay? In that statement, Kong Le made a sharp break with his previous moderate remarks on the subject of the Pathet Lao and declared that they were seeking "to make the Kingdom of Laos a new kind of colony of international communism." He went on to contend that the communist aim was to use Laos as the base from which they planned "to spread their evil policy." If young Corporal Kong had known of Kong Le's remarks, if he had come to believe that the man he was guarding was endangering his kingdom, we have perhaps found the motivation for the assassination.

◆ ◆ ◆

As the Mekong courses south, below Pakse, below Champassak, just before it reaches Cambodia, it divides for a few miles to flow past a lovely, verdant strip of land: Khong Island, the fief of the mandarin Abhay family.

I spent a day there when we were marking the completion of some public works—roads and an addition to the medical clinic— that had been accomplished by USAID. Our visit was in the nature of a celebration: ribbon cutting, speeches, and a festive buffet. Khong Island, as one wandered about, was seductive. The *wats* and houses were exceptionally trim, the rice fields and farms were neatly arranged, and even the minute airport had an efficient and cheerful air. Tropical trees in various green covered much of the land that had not been cultivated. It was easy to understand why the Abhays, although established as one of the important families in Vientiane, were always under the spell of their island home.

Nhouy Abhay was the shining intellectual of the family. His brother, Kou Abhay, was a patrician figure who early in 1960 had served for several months as provisional prime minister. Kouprasith Abhay, Nhouy's nephew, was eventually to become the head of the Lao armies and as such play a role in a later part of this history. But when I was in Vientiane in 1963, Nhouy became a special friend.

A singularly learned man, he could have taught French litera- ture in French but preferred to be the most notable scholar of Lao literature in Laos. He served at one time as Lao minister of education. When the French cultural review, *France-Asie,* in 1956 prepared its special edition on Laos, Nhouy was asked to write the chapters on Buddhism, festivals, rites, versification in Lao poetry, and the epic poem *Sin Xay.*

To suggest his witty, humanistic erudition, I cite two sentences selected almost at random from his article on versification: "After what has just been said about the material structure of Lao verse, one might be tempted to suppose it presents all the monotonous characteristics of which the classical French alexandrine was once accused, for it always falls into two hemistiches whose rhythm is 3 + 4 or 5 + 4. This is not, however, the case, and a Lao poem is as varied from the point of view of metre and rhythm as a romantic poem."

I first met Nhouy at one of those innumerable Vientiane receptions. Although fighting continued and the little kingdom lived under a threatening cloud, social life in Vientiane was intense, a never-ending cascade of cocktail and dinner parties. Members of the diplomatic corps, Lao officials, and certain prominent Lao figures met and remet at these gatherings. When I encountered Nhouy, I realized that even in a crowded room or garden he had something to say that was worth hearing and was amusing.

My memory of this man remains focused on a series of four or five tête-à-têtes, which came about as a result of telephone calls he made to my office. "Perry, what are you doing? Come by, I want to see you." I went by.

Nhouy's house was a throwback to an earlier Vientiane. Although located near the embassy, it seemed out of the city. To reach it, one passed an ancient *stupa* of graceful shape, some twenty feet in height. At a short distance beyond this monument, one entered an unexpected pastoral setting with a large field populated by several placid buffalo. Of the few houses located there, the first on the left was the largest, and this was Nhouy's. In true village fashion it rested on poles, its front a long veranda covered by a swooping overhang of a roof.

When I arrived, Nhouy would be waiting on the porch to greet me with warm salutations. He was a wizened creature with eyes sunken well into his skull but nevertheless brightly shining. Unlike most of his fellow countrymen, he looked old—older than his age.

The floors of the wooden porch buckled slightly, and the rattan chairs needed mending, but this was genteel neglect, not poverty. We would sit on that veranda with a table between us on which would be crystal glasses, soda, and a bottle of Johnny Walker. A disheveled servant came out periodically with a few melting ice cubes in a magnificent large silver bowl. Nhouy poured stiff drinks for both of us.

He was an alcoholic. He loved his whiskey and drank it excessively. Eventually it killed him, as I am sure he knew it would. Sometimes as we spoke he grew a bit incoherent or sleepy and I would leave so that he could return to his bed.

I remember quite precisely some of his remarks. With apologies to the memory of a man whose superb command of the French language and incisive wit are difficult even to approximate, I have attempted to reconstitute one of those conversations.

Nhouy: My young friend, do you enjoy being in Vientiane?

Perry: Definitely.

Nhouy: Why?

Perry: You have such beautiful women.

Nhouy: An excellent reason. Pretty girls—and music—and elephants—we have those in abundance. I wonder if we shall survive.

Perry: You are always pessimistic, Excellency.

Nhouy: You Americans are far too optimistic. I am an Asian educated in France—dire predictions come easily to me. Idealism could have been conceived of only by an Englishman. No Frenchman would be caught dead with that as a philosophy. But you Americans are imbued with it, even your pragmatism is idealistic. And this leads you to believe that virtue, which you equate with democracy, must triumph.

Perry: No, we're not saying that. We are trying to coexist with communism.

Nhouy: And I say that in the back of your minds, you are convinced that when the communists realize the joys of capitalism they will give up their system for yours. But I don't think you're going to be able to contain communism—not in our time. You're simply not tough enough.

A few moments later:

Nhouy: Did you attend the prime minister's press conference yesterday?

Perry: I did.

Nhouy: You heard him extol neutrality. Do you believe in this neutrality of ours?

Perry: Yes, don't you?

Nhouy: (After a long swig of his drink) No.

Perry: No, Excellency?

Nhouy: No. The prince thinks it wise not to choose between the materialistic corruption of the right and the perverted idealism of the left. Note that the communists, too, pay verbal tribute to idealism. But the prince is wrong. No man, no nation, can remain in the middle.

Perry: It seems to me that neutrality is the only policy that gives Laos a chance. Would you prefer to have General Phoumi stay at the head of your government?

Nhouy: Certainly, even though I'm not a Phoumi man.

Perry: (Smiling) Why aren't you, Excellency?

Nhouy: Let us admit that none of us with property and servants can be deemed wholly above corruption, but Phoumi started his life with neither property nor servants and has become extremely greedy. He began his career, as you know, as an enlisted man in the French army. No wonder he hates the French. Yet he has the ambition, force, guile, charisma to be the leader of the right, and as such he has been fairly successful.

Perry: Successful? Certainly not as a military leader.

Nhouy: True, he has never known what to do with an army. Military strategy is not his forte. Do you know him well?

Perry: When living in Savannakhet, I saw him a good many times, but no, I know him only slightly.

Nhouy: I am sure you do not like him. And do you know Prince Souvanna Phouma?

Perry: I have met him only briefly on several occasions.

Nhouy: And you admire him?

Perry: Enormously.

Nhouy: That follows. Souvanna is a gentleman and honorable—and dangerous.

Perry: Why dangerous?

Nhouy: He is unable to recognize the hypocrisy that prevails. But those of us on the right deceive ourselves less than do our cousins on the left. They pretend to be solely concerned with the well-being of the masses, a pretext they use to increase their personal power and wealth. We on the other side can admit, even if reluctantly, that we care primarily for ourselves. I admit that I enjoy wealth—I don't want to be deprived of my whiskey. And yet, my young friend, we are all victims, all without exception, and our choice is limited. I prefer to capitulate to capitalism. Souvanna will eventually have to make the same choice.

❈ ❈ ❈

Diplomacy is such a subtle art that its foremost practitioners are effective quietly, unobtrusively. Rarely do we have an example of an outstanding diplomat whose actions gain immediate, positive, splashy results.

On April 24, 1963, President Kennedy held a press conference, a good portion of which was devoted to Laos. The little kingdom was again on the front pages, for the situation on the Plain of Jars was not just bad, it was deteriorating. The Pathet Lao–North Vietnamese armies now menaced the neutralists to an even greater degree. The Chinese, competing fiercely for the affection of the North Vietnamese, had declared that the Russians were not sufficiently supportive of the Asian communists. To defuse the Chinese outbursts, the Soviets charged that the Plain of Jars confrontation was the result of interference by the United States.

The president, in answer to a question, said:

> The struggle is not between the forces of Phoumi [Nosavan] and the neutralists but between the Pathet Lao and the Kong Le forces, which, of course, are the army of Souvanna Phouma, whom the communists themselves supported in 1961. So I think we have a very clear idea where the responsibility lies, and it would be a distortion to place the breakdown upon the United States. . . . Now the solution is not to engage in polemics or debate but to bring about a cease-fire and to see if we can maintain what is a very fragile structure today.

Kennedy announced that on the following day Averell Harriman would be going to Moscow to confer with Foreign Minister Andrei Gromyko on the worsening situation in Laos.

News of the president's assignment reached Harriman while he was in London, conferring about Laos with the British foreign secretary, the Earl of Home. Governor Harriman, that debonair aristocrat, heir to a vast fortune, polo player turned political luminary, former governor of New York, former ambassador to the Soviet Union, was enjoying the role for which his life had richly prepared him—diplomat *extraordinaire.* He terminated his visit to London and flew directly to Moscow.

Details play a special importance in diplomatic protocol, and the welcome he received on this occasion signaled impending defeat. A person of his rank and prominence coming with a personal message from the president had to be met officially at the airport by no one less than a deputy foreign minister. When Harriman disembarked from the plane, a lowly deputy chief of protocol was there to represent the Soviet government—a deliberate snub. And when Harriman asked at what time the next day he was to meet with Gromyko, the reply was that no time had been set.

Rather than feeling sensitive about this rebuff, the governor took the matter in stride and set about arranging details in his own manner. And so the following day, Harriman met not with Gromyko but with Premier Khrushchev himself. Even more remarkable was that the meeting between the two men became an intense discussion which lasted for three and a half hours. At the conclusion, this statement, drafted in Russian, was issued: "The President [of the United States] and the [Soviet] Chairman of the Council of Ministers reaffirmed that both governments fully support the Geneva agreement on Laos," Mission accomplished, the governor returned to Washington.

Some critics carped that this statement failed to assure Moscow's intervention vis-à-vis the North Vietnamese–Pathet Lao troops to halt the fighting on the Plain of Jars. However, I can think of no other person President Kennedy could have sent to Moscow under those circumstances who could have engaged Khrushchev in a long talk on the situation and who could have come out of it with positive support for the Lao government.

Averell Harriman was, simply, and clearly, a great diplomat.

❋ ❋ ❋

Viewed from afar and within a specific time frame, a nation's history has its beginnings, its development, and its resultant state. Laos gaining its independence from the French, or the little kingdom having its neutrality established by the Geneva conference, might be considered beginnings that held promise— tenuous promise to be sure. But rather than develop, the unfortunate kingdom then lurched on to tragedy. History as it was experienced in Laos was a condition of unremitting intensity and countless crises.

The International Control Commission that the wise men of Geneva had created to oversee the kingdom's neutrality was constantly challenged. A few weeks after Harriman's visit to Moscow, the commission came to partial grief on one of those infrequent occasions when the three chief commissioners were acting in accord.

A group of French missionaries was stranded in the northern town of Xiengkhouang. My year in Savannakhet revealed to me that missionaries may be expected to be found virtually anywhere. Xiengkhouang was definitely not the place they should have been. The town had fallen under Pathet Lao control, but the nearby Meo hill tribes were not accepting this Pathet Lao incursion and were fighting it. These missionaries were caught in the middle. For several weeks they had been stranded in this minor but bloody battle zone until efforts finally prevailed to have them evacuated by road. They left the besieged town, but one of the trucks transporting them hit a land mine. Many were injured, and a French sergeant was killed.

The International Control Commission agreed to investigate. A principal resource of the commission had been four helicopters that allowed the commissioners the mobility necessary to conduct their investigative functions. Two months previously, one chopper had had engine trouble and made an emergency landing on Pathet Lao territory. Before the mechanics from Vientiane could get to the scene, it had been stripped beyond hope of salvage. That left three helicopters.

The missionaries' misfortune was the cause of international consternation in Vientiane, and when the three chief commissioners set off for the Xiengkhouang site, the prime minister, the British ambassador and the French first secretary accompanied them. Two of the remaining choppers were recruited to carry this notable group of passengers.

The aircrafts arrived at their destination. Shortly after the passengers debarked and left the landing field, a contingent of Pathet Lao soldiers bombarded the helicopters with shells that destroyed both of them. There were no casualties, but the feeble commission was made even weaker, and it would take time and major new funds to replace the vital means of transportation.

The prime minister returned to Vientiane furious and frustrated, and the war tumbled on.

◆ ◆ ◆

In a city in which many diplomats reside, the political and military situations may be grim, but the plethora of receptions and dinner parties will never cease. During 1963, when the neutralist government was being so sorely tried, social life in Vientiane was most agreeable.

I enjoyed this year in the little kingdom's capital not only for the party syndrome, in such marked contrast to Savannakhet, but also because of the Americans who now made up the Information Agency. The public affairs officer was Gerry Gert, a refugee from Germany who had come to America, served in the army, graduated from a university, and developed into a fine foreign service officer. His deputy, John Stoddard, a Princetonian from New England, seemed simply too kind to be an effective leader but proved himself to be a strong if amiable one. John and his charming wife Jean are an utterly delightful couple. Håkon Torjesen and his wife Karen are of Norwegian missionary background, and she, a young medical doctor, worked as a volunteer at the orphanage of the local hospital. Before the Torjesens left Laos for Africa, they adopted from the orphanage a baby girl whom Karen was nursing to health and who of course became equally as important a member of the family as their two very blonde children. More recently, all of the Torjesens, parents and children, left their home in Minneapolis to spend half a year at a Lao refugee camp in Thailand.

The American ambassador was Leonard Unger, a career diplomat par excellence. He and his lovely wife Anne and their children integrated themselves beautifully into the Lao scene.

That year the Lao Red Cross chose to have for its annual fund-raising event a performance at the Ecole Natasinh. The embassies were urged to participate in the evening's entertainment, and participate we did. For weeks, ten of us, including Anne Unger, her daughter Debbie, and John and Jean Stoddard, took off time at the end of each day's work to rehearse strenuously before proceeding on to our evening activities. A staff member of the American embassy knew her choreography and put us through our paces in a chorus line routine which concluded with an exuberant Charleston. We acquired gaudy costumes for the event, and when Anne Unger appeared at the dress rehearsal in a beguiling flapper-type wig, one embassy officer chatted with her without recognizing her. We thought our dance was the hit of the Red Cross evening, but that my have been because we so much enjoyed going through our steps and hamming it up before a large audience.

But back to work—back to my job.

The role of an American ambassador is to help carry out foreign policy formulated by the president and the secretary of state. The ambassador needs to be extraordinarily well informed in order to advise, but he should not make or pronounce new policy. In one instance, I instigated a certain violation of the principle. Here is how it happened. The morning market was a remarkably colorful sight. This huge, open compound on the Avenue Lan Xang, between the river and the government circle, was the focal point each morning of enormous activity. Vendors, mostly of food, prepared their wares well before sunrise, and until noon countless people came to look and buy. More than a hundred pedicabs would line up on the avenue to provide transportation.

Many a foreigner would be intimidated by the idea of making his way through the old market. There was a scheme to the arrangements, but it was difficult to divine. Stalls were packed tightly, aisles were too narrow and encumbered, meats, poultry, fish, and overripe fruit had minimal or no refrigeration—all factors blunting the appeal of the often exotic produce. The Lao themselves had begun to complain about the condition and the inability of the mart to cope with the increasing population.

USAID wisely offered to undertake a complete restructuring of the morning market. The offer was readily accepted by the government and handsomely carried out at considerable expense. New and extensive refrigeration facilities were installed, and the meat and fish areas were separated by at least a wide aisle from the fruits, vegetables, and sundries. The aesthetic aspects were more than respected—they were enhanced. A majestic, gigantic new roof was constructed in traditional Lao style, its tiers sharply sloping down and then turning upward with graceful corners rivaling those of the temples.

When the work was completed, an inaugural ceremony was scheduled, and I was given the assignment of drafting the Ambassador's speech. We were still in the early post-Geneva period, and although it was more than evident that the Pathet Lao incursions were as ongoing as though the Geneva conference had never taken place, in official remarks we continued to laud the recently established neutralist government rather than to denounce the Pathet Lao—or the rightists—for grievous infractions of the accords. It was therefore expected that the ambassador's talk would adhere to this policy.

But try as I might, I could not come up with the good will remarks that such an occasion was expected to call forth. The situation on the Plain of Jars was too grave for that, and it was foolhardy to pretend that the little kingdom was not in danger. After many attempts and many torn up sheets of paper, I wrote a strong rebuke to the Pathet Lao. I played with it, made unsuccessful efforts to soften it, and finally, somewhat sheepishly, showed it to the ambassador. He read it, agreed with it, and made only a few minor changes.

The day of the inauguration was a festive one. A large turnout of officials and diplomats filled the temporary stands, and crowds gathered in front of the impressive new morning market. Len Unger rose to the podium and read his speech. It was listened to and politely applauded. And that, we thought, was that.

We were wrong. The speech, which had been meant for local

consumption, was picked up everywhere. *The New York Times* gave it prominence, and the Associated Press in its dispatch sent out worldwide called the attack against the Pathet Lao "a minor diplomatic bombshell."

I was troubled to think that Len Unger might be called upon to account for his remarks, but I was, I admit, somewhat amused to have been partially responsible for a diplomatic bombshell, albeit a minor one.

◆ ◆ ◆

At home when I was a growing lad, we used to play an occasional game of bridge—my father, my sister, and whoever we could inveigle into being a fourth. Ours was more a game of intuition—of trying to read your opponent's and partner's minds—than of logic and rules. It tended to be emotional, but it was fun.

I seldom played the game again until the war years—my war, World War II—when I was an ensign at Cockspur Island Naval Base in Georgia. The officers stationed on the island were allowed to "go ashore"—meaning to nearby Savannah—every other night, but that left the long nights in between at the oh-so-quiet BOQ—Bachelor Officers Quarters. It so happened that three senior officers at the base were exceptionally good bridge players, and they were in need of a fourth body, anyone who knew the basic rules. I was content to be their man, and after many sessions of getting drubbed, I began to play a competitive game. When I left Cockspur and indulged in the game elsewhere, I learned that I had become quite a proficient bridger.

Through the ensuing years I would get involved with fellow players, but then there would be arid stretches of abstinence. However, I consistently maintained an interest and enthusiasm and still read religiously the bridge hand in every newspaper I fall upon.

I write of this because being a bridge player made an enormous difference in my life. In Vientiane I played with certain members of the French mission. One of them, René Weill, a most witty man who ran the French-language radio programs for the Lao government, was friend of the prime minister. It was common knowledge in diplomatic circles that Prince Souvanna Phouma was a passionate bridge player. René played with him often, and one day René invited me to spend an evening at the prime minister's residence. Fresh blood was wanted at the table, and I was to provide it.

As we were leaving the office that afternoon, Håkon asked if I had any plans for the evening. I replied that as a matter of fact, I did: I was going to have dinner and play bridge with the prime minister. Håkon hooted: "Stieglitz, you can't do that. You're only a junior officer."

The sentry at the gate recognized René's car and casually saluted as we drove past on the curved pebbled driveway to the prime minister's two-storied, white stucco French colonial house. From the entrance hall we stepped into the salon, a long tall room whose height was emphasized by several pairs of columns. Crystal chandeliers hung from the ceiling. At one end of the room, doors led into the prime minister's offices, and at the other end was the library. The furnishings throughout were in an impeccable French style adapted to the tropical climate.

The prince received us cordially. We had drinks and chatted, touching on both international and personal matters. There was an exceptional aura about Souvanna Phouma. He seemed to epitomize so many fine qualities—knowledge and intelligence, sensitivity, strength without arrogance—that I thought him to be the most civilized man I had ever met. I still hold to that opinion.

His only other guest that evening was Henri Cotin, a longtime French adviser to the Lao government who worked largely with the prime minister's affairs. Henri was a white-haired, soft-spoken gentleman who had lived for many years in the little kingdom with his Lao wife and children. I had met him previously, had played cards with him, and enjoyed his company.

Not long after we arrived, our host announced: "*Messieurs, à table.*" He did not mean the dining table. It was too early for that. We proceeded to the bridge table.

The prince was a brilliant player. After two or three discards, he seemed to know precisely which cards remained in which hands, and he used this knowledge to excellent advantage. It was not easy to be his partner, for he was exigent. If you misplayed, he was apt to comment, but not discourteously. Nevertheless, I remember one evening the wife of a diplomat who was the prince's partner for a rubber suddenly crying out: "*Altesee,* I'm too nervous to play with you." But he was generous in his compliments to both partners and opponents.

That first evening, the four of us played for a while and then went into the dining room, which had been added on to the house by the prince. The room could accommodate thirty-six persons for an official dinner, and it was also used for cabinet meetings. A long room, it sustained perfectly the style of the house. One must not forget that Souvanna Phouma was an architect.

We ate well, an unusual combination of Asian and French dishes served not together but in turn and drank a good wine, but it was understood that this was merely a prelude to a return to the card table. There we drank coffee and fine Cognac and smoked hefty Havanas—these latter tend to make me feel slightly intoxicated.

The gods were with me: I played well. I will not make the banal suggestion that I was lucky and held good cards. When playing with an expert, good or poor cards mean little. When the session ended long after midnight, I was led to understand that I had been accepted as a member of the prime minister's bridge club, and I was thankful to those three naval officers who had forced upon me the necessary training.

I might remark that at the prince's house bridge was played for no stakes or minimal ones. When he played poker, which he also enjoyed, it was for moderate stakes.

Afterward, when I would encounter Prince Souvanna at receptions or dinner parties, he was most cordial. I was invited to his residence for small games or large dinners. It was traditional that after the meal had been served and the guests were having their coffee and liqueurs the moment would come when the prince would announce: "*Mesdames, messieurs, à table.*" Those who were to play, and they knew in advance who they were, would move on to the card tables. The other guests—they might be ambassadors or cabinet members—would remain in the salon for further conversation or another drink if they chose, and then they would depart without interrupting the contest in the next room, a contest that often continued late into the night.

In using all of his statesmanship and political skills on behalf of his country, Souvanna Phouma found respite in employing other, perhaps similar skills at the game of bridge.

The advent of the wet season failed to change the little kingdom's overall situation. The Pathet Lao, urged on by the physical presence of the North Vietnamese armies, continued their military advances while the resentful rightists under Phoumi Nosavan, still hopeful for regaining full command, obstructed progress. Both factions acknowledged that Souvanna Phouma was the country's natural leader, but many did so grudgingly.

In November, among the official visitors from Washington was my old friend, Michelle. Her last tour in Vientiane had been abruptly abrogated in early 1962, not long after the Battle of Vientiane, when Phoumi had usurped the government. The American ambassador had never been happy with the outspoken Michelle, and since she had been an ardent partisan of Souvanna Phouma and the prince was in exile, the ambassador used this as an opportunity to rid himself of her. With great sorrow, she left the little kingdom.

She had been thrilled by the change of administrations in Washington—by the replacement of J. Graham Parsons—and most of all by President Kennedy sending Averell Harriman to be his envoy to Southeast Asia. Michelle felt certain that Harriman and Souvanna would appreciate each other, and she was not at all surprised that their relationship brought about the change she had advocated in the American posture toward the little kingdom. Back at work in the State Department, she brought as much support as she could to the neutralist Lao government.

When she returned to Vientiane in November of 1963, she was delighted to be warmly welcomed by many, many Lao friends. She was also pleased that the American Fulbright grantee she had tutored in the ways and politics of the country was now attached to the embassy.

Thanksgiving was approaching, and I suggested that she who had entertained in this city so often and so significantly might care to invite a few of her friends for a holiday dinner at my small house. She pounced upon the idea. The next day, quivering with excitement, she told me that the prime minister was going to have Thanksgiving dinner with us.

"He is?" I asked.

She smiled triumphantly.

Within days, the most wrenching piece of public news in a

lifetime struck: John F. Kennedy had been assassinated. Some of us feared—and with reason—that this unthinkable event would have terrible consequences for Southeast Asia. Memorial services were held in the royal temple in Vientiane, and it seemed that everyone, from the king to pedicab drivers, mourned this foreign leader who had played a major—and I believe entirely beneficial—role in the history of the little kingdom.

Thanksgiving dinner was celebrated solemnly. Because Prince Souvanna was attending, other luminaries had also been invited, making it all somewhat big for the cottage's britches. To complete the evening, though, we did play bridge.

In the Foreign Service, you spend two years at a post, and you become accustomed to the house in which you live and the culture which surrounds you. Then one day a cable comes in and announces that you are to leave for some perhaps totally unexpected post where you will have to create immediately upon arrival your new existence. This pattern might be traumatic for most people, but for many of us in the service, it enriched our lives.

In December 1963, my cable came and announced that I was assigned to Paris as assistant cultural affairs officer. I let out a howl of joy, and for days, friends and I were in a nonstop celebration of my good fortune. No other post could have pleased me more.

While making preparations to leave, I asked at the prime minister's office if I might call to say goodbye, and an appointment was promptly given to me.

We sat in his office, Prince Souvanna and I. Despite my happiness, I was genuinely sad to be taking leave of this extraordinary man and of his country, to which I had grown so devoted. He had heard about my assignment and congratulated me. We spoke about Paris—the city where he had earned his degree as an architect, the city where he had served as ambassador.

"*Altesse*," I inquired, "what can I do for you while I am there?"

"Nothing," he replied. Then he reflected and declared: "Yes, there is something. Once in a while, look after my children."

III

Paris: Three Princes, Two Princesses
1964–1967

In Laos, during my year in Savannakhet, I had been a field officer. In France, I again was a field officer. Shortly after I had arrived in Paris in January of 1964, Lee Brady, the public affairs officer, called me into his office and informed me that he was about to give me the best of all possible assignments. And he did. I was put in charge of our cultural and informational programs throughout the country outside of Paris. To carry out my mission, I traveled by auto, train, and plane to all corners of that magnificent land. Consequently, I grew to know it in a way that few ever do. Every gothic cathedral and many of the Romanesque churches became familiar to me, and every two- and three-star restaurant was at least sampled. Since those years, it sometimes happens that I will be chatting with a Frenchman who speaks of some cherished spot that is, he is happy to relate, *bien caché*, but when I am able to describe it in detail, he is apt to resent this foreigner's transgression of his domain.

My cake had several layers of icing. Within days of my arrival, I was fortunate to find an ideal apartment. A distinguished French literary agent, Marguerite Scialtiel, sent me to see a flat that another of her friends was about to vacate. A quick glimpse was all that was necessary. A small but spacious Art Deco duplex on the corner of the Avenue Victor Hugo and Rue Saint Didier, its personality was evoked by an American of a certain age who looked about and then, pointing to the staircase that led up to the bedroom, demanded: "When does Constance Bennett come down those stairs?"

After several unsuccessful tries to find household help, a heavy-set, fierce, and entirely remarkable Burgundian woman came to the apartment to interview me, and a demanding interview it was. Gabrielle did not care much for Americans, but two factors were in my favor: she lived nearby, and she would be able to take charge in the way only a bachelor would tolerate. So she became *ma gouvernante*. Helen McCully, the food editor of *House Beautiful*, came to dinner and declared Gabrielle's soufflé to be unsurpassable.

When I was not on the road, life in Paris was, as one might expect, crowded with enticing activities. There were the theaters and the concerts and the art galleries. On some evenings when they were not performing, I would see a certain French actress who was featured in a boulevard comedy or another who was in the repertoire of the Comédie Francaise.

Our ambassador was that outstanding diplomat Charles Bohlen. As an available bachelor, I would, if in town, occasionally receive a telephone call from Mrs. Bohlen's social secretary telling me to be at the residence in black tie that evening to replace at the table an ailing guest. In this way, I sat in for some notable Frenchmen.

Averell Harriman was at the embassy in Paris for several days in early spring. I had never met the governor and was very surprised to be told that he wished to see me. When I entered the small office he was temporarily occupying, he was sitting at the desk, but his tall imposing presence filled the room. Everyone in the Foreign Service had heard stories about his tremendous accomplishments and amusing peccadillos, but only as I sat there on the opposite side of the desk could I realize how keen was his mind, how considerate his nature.

He had a strong attachment to Laos and had informed himself thoroughly on the subject, even in minor details. In this way, he had come to know about me. I was embarrassed and touched to hear him thank me for any concern for the little kingdom. Then he went on to speak of young Prince Panya Souvanna Phouma, who was completing his studies at the Ecole des Hautes Etudes Commerciales in Paris and wished to go on to Harvard Business School. The governor was going to arrange this, but there were certain forms to be filled out and some other details for which I could be of assistance, and he asked me to undertake this task.

Panya, therefore, was the first of Prince Souvanna's children whom I tried to look after.

The young prince came to see me at my office. He was remarkably handsome, of good height, and solidly athletic. He was a rugby player and would become captain of the rugby team at Harvard Business School. He was also outgoing and charming, displaying all of the finesse one would hope that a young man with his inheritance would possess.

I had seen Princess Souvanna Phouma on only a few occasions in Vientiane, for her position as director of international organizations with the Lao Ministry of Foreign Affairs kept here largely in Europe, where she represented her country at meetings of UNESCO, World Health, Food and Agriculture, and other organizations. As a result of my helping Panya, I saw her more often in France.

The princess was the prototype of a grande dame. A large woman with regal bearing, she was deeply serious in her work with the United Nations and expressed herself eloquently on behalf of the kingdom. Her manner was warm and friendly but with a certain reserve. She was extraordinarily elegant, and her beautifully decorated Paris apartment was always filled with huge vases of flowers. The title *Altesse* perfectly became her. Later that spring, Ambassador and Mrs. Bohlen held a dinner party for the princess and Panya, and I was one of the few Americans present, an arrangement, I suspect, that may have been suggested by the governor.

Its continuing crises plus the enveloping Vietnamese war kept Laos prominent in the international news. The French, who had treated Laos poorly when it was their colony, now regarded it as a *cause célèbre*.

And I who had said farewell to the little kingdom when I left Vientiane learned that my ties to it would be strengthened rather than diminished while I was in France.

❀ ❀ ❀

The three political factions of Laos, each headed by a prince, would never, it had seemed, be able to resolve their basic differences, but the efforts they made to do so were, I found, fascinating. In April of 1964, they selected as the site of a reunion a tent on the disputed Plain of Jars in the northern part of the kingdom. This meeting brought them as close to an agreement as they would ever be and was in its physical arrangements unique, dramatic, and amusing.

To allay the mutual suspicions of Prince Souphanouvong and of General Phoumi Nosavan, who acted as a substitute for Prince Boun Oum, these were the conditions: outside the tent were posted three bodyguards—one for each—and six servants—two for each. Measured from the tent by a radius of fifty yards was a circle manned by thirty unarmed soldiers—ten for each. And beyond that circle, fifty yards farther, was another circle, this one occupied by three hundred soldiers—yes, one hundred for each. How extraordinary it might have been from the vantage view of a hovering helicopter to have looked down upon this military spectacle staged in the style of Busby Berkeley.

Prince Souvanna Phouma and Phoumi arrived on the scene from Vientiane, but separately. Souphanouvong came down from the north. The two princes were dashingly attired in fine summer suits. Souvanna sported a homburg and large pearl stickpin in his cravat. The general wore fatigues.

The three entered the tent on the morning of the seventeenth, paused for a good box lunch brought up from Vientiane, continued the session in the afternoon, and then adjourned for the day. The press was permitted to approach and ask questions. Prince Souvanna said: "Our points of view were quite close to each other," and added that he hoped the next day would bring "concrete results." Prince Souphanouvong declared himself to be optimistic. And General Phoumi surprised the newsmen when he remarked that he was encouraged and that the meeting had been held in a "cordial atmosphere."

Some might have assumed that peace was at hand. Unfortunately, that assumption led to another event, one that had enormous influence on the kingdom.

General Siho Lamphouthacoul, formerly Colonel Siho, the henchman of Phoumi Nosavan in the days when Phoumi was rising in power, had himself risen in rank to an important directorship of the quasi-military police department in Vientiane. Siho's background, about which Seymour Topping wrote a fine story of detection and insight for *The New York Times*, is important to these events of April 1964. Siho was born on lovely Khong Island, the fief of the mandarin Abhay family. His Chinese-Lao parents were employed in the household of Kou Abhay. Kouprasith Abhay, Kou's eldest son, was ten years older than Siho, and Siho claimed that Kouprasith had treated him badly. Just how badly we can only conjecture. Was it the haughty manner of a spoiled mandarin's son toward a servant in the house, or was it a more calculated cruelty? Whatever it was, the inordinately ambitious Siho was strongly resentful of Kouprasith.

Siho studied at the Lao military academy and later at a military training college in France. He was disliked and feared by most of the Lao, but Phoumi made him a protégé and had him appointed director of national coordination, giving the young man tremendous power. And he used that power ruthlessly.

Siho went to Taiwan in 1963 for advanced general staff training and while there came under the influence of the director of the Chinese national security services, General Chiang Ching-kuo, son of Chiang Kai-shek. But Siho hardly seemed to need such training for he had already introduced infamous police methods, including torture, into the little kingdom.

General Kouprasith was in 1964 the military commander of Vientiane. He was a large, paunchy man who could at times be testy and at other times appeared to lack dedicated ambition and political commitment. It was widely assumed that the Abhay name had gained for him his eminent position.

Siho, an extreme rightist, politically and economically naive, was disgruntled with the Geneva accords and the tripartite government. He drew Kouprasith and certain other officers into a conspiracy with the intention of overthrowing the government. He argued that when they took over, the United States would have no choice but to accept them and support them, just as the United States had supported Phoumi in the Battle of Vientiane. On April 17, the optimistic reports that emanated from the meeting of the princes on the Plain of Jars forced Siho's hand.

Souvanna Phouma, Souphanouvong, and Phoumi met again in their well-guarded tent on the Plain of Jars on the morning of the eighteenth. This session broke up after only two hours with totally negative results, and the three went their separate ways. Prince Souvanna returned to Vientiane and announced that he was considering resigning.

The danger that Siho feared—a peace of sorts among the three factions—had vanished, but the countdown for his coup had begun and was not to be turned off. He was relieved that his mentor, Phoumi, was out of town. Phoumi had not been consulted on this action. As for Kouprasith, Siho could not really trust the man, and so he locked him up in Kouprasith's own apartment at Camp Chinaimo, their military headquarters.

By five the next morning, a Sunday, Siho's troops raced through the city and shot a few soldiers who opposed them. The prime minister's residence was encircled, and the prince was informed that he was under house arrest. Other leading neutralists' homes were surrounded. Within an hour, this rightist rebel group controlled the airport, the radio station, the city. An announcement was made that the Revolutionary Committee of the National Army was in charge and that the committee was, in a classic example of hiding behind a front, headed by General Kouprasith. Siho was named second in command.

For many of us, it was difficult to take this with the gravity that a *coup d'état* usually demands. Except for those half dozen soldiers who were unfortunate enough to be shot, this coup had a somewhat comic air. One could hardly imagine Siho as head of state. Nor could one readily picture Kouprasith in that role, and his reputation was not helped when we learned that he had ludicrously been a prisoner when the coup took place in his name. However, for a world increasingly alarmed about Southeast Asian affairs and therefore concerned about the little kingdom, Siho's coup earned for two successive days three-column headlines as the lead story on *The New York Times'* front page. That newspaper's editorial, though, did reflect a certain cynicism in its heading, "Laos Falls Apart Again."

In the crisis, quiet, smiling, soft-spoken Ambassador Leonard Unger's derring-do was outstanding. He was conferring with Secretary of State Dean Rusk in Saigon when the coup occurred, and Unger returned at once to Vientiane. He proceeded directly to Camp Chinaimo, where the gates and doors were closed to him. That did not deter him. He pushed all barriers aside until he was face to face with the junta masters, Siho and Kouprasith. He told them in absolute terms that the United States fully supported the Geneva accords and that the junta could count on no recognition, no aid from America. Siho was furious, and Kouprasith began to understand more fully the folly in which he was engaged.

Unger went from Camp Chinaimo to the prime minister's residence. The soldiers were massed about it, and no one was permitted to pass through their lines. Len Unger was undaunted. He went through, made his way to the residence, stood beneath the balcony of the prime minister's bedroom, and read as loudly as his voice would carry the contents of a letter he had with him. The letter was an official document declaring the full support of the United States government for Souvanna Phouma and his neutralist government. As he was reading this, the doors of the balcony opened, Souvanna stepped out, smiled down, and the two men exchanged greetings and remarks of assurance. If the soldiers who witnessed this had been familiar with English literature, they might have made comparisons with the Bard's balcony scene.

Kouprasith and Siho flew to Luang Prabang to present their new government to the king. They were convinced that he would approve their having rid the government of its communist elements. To their dismay, His Majesty chastised them in the harshest terms. It is reported that Kouprasith broke down and wept, while Siho's resentment against the world grew. The two generals returned to Vientiane but, at Siho's insistence, did not relinquish their new power.

Then yet another extraordinary event happened in the kingdom, a most remarkable manifestation of international unity: the ambassadors of the United States, the Soviet Union, Britain, France, Australia, and India flew up to Luang Prabang for an audience with the king. They urged him to reject the coup and to return the government to Souvanna Phouma. It was evident that the king was sympathetic to their cause even before they expressed it.

And His Majesty evinced his own worldliness on this occasion. When a statement drawn up by the ambassadors was read, it began with a disclaimer to any wish to interfere in the internal affairs of Laos. When the king heard that, he laughed and exclaimed: *"Vraiment?"*

Siho's coup did not end with any finality; rather it withered away. But it had several long-term results. Because Siho and Kouprasith had acted without Phoumi Nosavan, a schism was rent in the rightists' camp, and Phoumi lost prestige among his followers. For Kouprasith, the coup was a severe and unforgettable embarrassment, but he was still relatively young, he had his family ties and wealth to sustain him, and he continued as a leading general of the Lao armies.

As for Siho Lamphouthacoul, his lifelong ambition and bitterness, his tutelage under such masters as Phoumi Nosavan and Chiang Ching-kuo, his innate brutality—all of these led to his moment of triumph when he controlled the country and the despised Kouprasith was at his bidding. Within days, his success had collapsed, and he was not merely a failure but an object of derision. It was gall and wormwood to know that Kouprasith would remain a mighty general whereas he, Siho, with no notable family, no wealth, no followers, faced ignominy.

The truism that being born into a privileged family is one of the greatest of assets may have been even more true in the little kingdom. Siho raged and blamed his fate on having been born into a family of servants rather than their masters. But Siho would once more be saved by his mentor, Phoumi Nosavan.

❋ ❋ ❋

This is the case of the recalcitrant Pole.

Marek Thee was the Polish chief commissioner of the International Control Commission. He wanted people to know that he came from an academic background. Former professors sometimes carry with them their classroom convictions that are untested outside the university walls, and when these academicians go into the diplomatic service they may forget that negotiations are the essence of diplomacy.

Undistinguished in appearance—medium height, medium weight, no remarkable facial characteristics—Thee was generally dour and made infrequent stabs at gaining social respectability. To this end, he once hosted a large Vientiane cocktail party at which ambassadors, ministers, and others were received by him with affected affability.

As a born-again communist, he was utterly dogmatic. As a loyal Pole, he did not wish to be thought of as subservient to the Russians. As a chief commissioner, he was an unholy terror.

It is hardly an exaggeration to believe that if the Pathet Lao had staged an attack a mile away from where he happened to be he would not only have refused to go to see the results but would have vetoed any ICC attempt to investigate. The Pathet Lao, according to Marek Thee, were never wrong. The rightists and the neutralists were capitalist warmongers.

The Geneva accords, which unfortunately depended upon the ICC and which compounded that error by expecting all ICC actions to be unanimous, became a cropper in the power it bestowed upon Thee.

In May of 1964, the Pathet Lao attacks on the Plain of Jars increased. Prince Souvanna Phouma requested that the ICC establish a permanent control group on the Plain. The Indian and Canadian commissioners readily agreed; Thee refused. Then he went beyond that and persuaded the Pathet Lao to withdraw their consent to the commission's presence.

Frustrations ran high. Counteractions were sought.

In 1963, the U.S. Congress had barred a most-favored-nation tariff treatment for Polish imports. The Kennedy administration had attempted to convince Congress to rescind that measure. But in May of 1964 the administration made it known to the Polish government that it would make no further efforts on Poland's behalf vis-à-vis the tariff if Thee continued to conduct himself in this unacceptable fashion. Thee was called back to Warsaw for consultations, and when he returned to Laos, he was slightly subdued.

Thus it happened that the behavior of a Polish official in the little kingdom almost changed the national policy of the United States toward Poland.

◆ ◆ ◆

The April summit had failed, but this did not discourage Prince Souvanna Phouma from his efforts to make the neutral tripartite government effective. By summertime he was arranging another get-together for the three princes with Paris as its site. It was hoped that France would provide a sympathetic climate for the discussions. I, of course, was delighted that it was going to take place in the city where I was.

In the two years since the accords had been signed in Geneva, the situation in Indochina had become far more complex. The Pathet Lao, always under North Vietnamese command, had violated the agreements and increased their military incursions, while the failed rightists' coup had aggravated further the discord within the kingdom. But it was the overall situation in the area that was the paramount concern in the negotiations of the major powers. Souvanna believed that the newly proposed summit should seek a reconvening of the fourteen-nation Geneva conference. The Soviets favored this idea, but the United States feared that the Russians would use such a forum to denounce American transgression in Vietnam and to demand neutralization of the entire area. Washington under Kennedy had come to support the neutralization of Laos—but only of Laos, not of Indochina. Washington's sensitivity on this point was heightened when President de Gaulle stated that France favored neutralization of all of Indochina. General de Gaulle predicted dire results if his advice was not heeded, and he tried to enlist Communist China on his side in the argument.

One morning in early August 1964, the public affairs officer called me into his office to tell me that although my field program was off to a fine start, he had been requested to remove me from it for a while in order to lend me to the embassy's political section for the duration of the meeting of the princes. The little kingdom had caught up with me again in a very big way.

So that there may be no disappointed expectations, let me say at once that the Paris summit failed to achieve any resolutions, failed as dismally as had the gathering in the tent on the Plain of Jars. But from my new involvement, I was able to be part of the Paris gathering and to have a close-up view of the Lao participants, most of whom seemed wonderfully impermeable to the pressures others tried to exert on them.

The State Department sent as the principal American observer Philip Chadbourn, a friend who had been deputy chief of mission in Vientiane. Philip is an amusing man. His father had a school in southern France, near Saint Tropez, when that was an unknown, sleepy Mediterranean village. Philip is completely bilingual and used his French to excellent advantage. He was a superior foreign service officer, and those who knew him well never doubted that he could have become a fine ambassador. But he never became one for he, like Prince Boun Oum, thought there was more to life than politics and international relations. After his retirement, Philip found his niche as an aide to Princess Grace and Prince Rainier in Monaco, where his exceptional charm was duly appreciated.

When he arrived in Paris that summer, he stayed in my apartment for a few days, which made life a bit crowded for both of us until he settled into his own hotel quarters. Then for the next six weeks we spent part of almost every day together—not unlike those detective teams who populate too many television serials and movies—and we, too, were trying to unravel a mystery, the mystery being precisely what was transpiring at the various sessions and what the prospects were for any substantive agreements.

Philip and I each had our knowledge of and insights into the assembled Lao personalities, and we would compare notes and attempt to assess their activities. We spent far too great a proportion of our time with the rightists, for they were most accessible to us; they welcomed our presence and urged us to eat with them at their favorite restaurant and to drink with them at their hotel and to play tennis with them. Philip was a popular figure with them and obviously enjoyed their company whereas I felt somewhat guilty because these men did not represent the team of my choice. The communists, as was to be expected, shunned us. I was able to see more of Prince Souvanna. The number two man of the neutralist delegation was Khampan Panya, a perplexing choice that we imagined had been imposed upon the delegation by the king: for Khampan, a close friend of His Majesty, was himself a strong rightist and spent much of his time in Paris in the company of the rightist delegates.

An announcement was made that no one other than members of the three delegations would be permitted to be present when the three princes met, and the first of such meetings was to take place on Monday, the twenty-fourth of August. The site, offered by the French government, was the handsome Château de la Celle Saint-Cloud on the outskirts of the city, but the Quai d'Orsay allowed it to be known, *sotto voce*, that they had not wanted the summit to take place in France unless they could be certain that the three factions would actually meet and not simply argue about meeting.

Here was the situation on Friday, August 21: Prince Souvanna Phouma arrived from Laos and made on optimistic statement. Prince Souphanouvong had not yet arrived, and no one could be found to give assurance that he would be there on time. Prince Boun Oum was out of town—he had gone to the Riviera. Ngon Sananikone, minister of public works, had accompanied Prince Souvanna to Paris, and it was believed that he would represent the rightists at the parley, for Phoumi Nosavan had stayed behind in Vientiane. Phoumi was deputy prime minister and was playing his favorite role as acting head of government in Souvanna's absence.

On Saturday, the Chinese Communist news agency announced that Prince Souphanouvong was on his way to Paris. The prince actually arrived on the evening of Tuesday, the twenty-fifth, the day after the summit was to have begun. On Wednesday, Prince Souvanna declared that the first meeting would "probably" be held on Friday. A new delay had been caused by Boun Oum's reluctance to attend, and three rightists delegates flew down to Nice to persuade their leader to lead.

Friday, the twenty-eighth, Souvanna and Souphanouvong held their first tête-à-tête. Following the Siho-Kouprasith coup, Souphanouvong, in the name of the Pathet Lao, had refused to recognize his half-brother's government as the legitimate government of the country, declaring it had become rightist dominated. Souphanouvong's assertion and the cease-fire upon which Souvanna insisted were the main points of discussion between the two princes.

Boun Oum relented and came up to Paris.

French Foreign Minister Couve de Murville held a dinner in honor of the three princes. At this dinner, the three were under the same roof in Paris for the first time that summer. The summit itself had not yet begun.

Prince Boun Oum remarked in public with a certain casualness that he was placing the rightists' negotiations in the hands of Souvanna Phouma. This complicated further the situation. Souphanouvong insisted Boun Oum's statement proved his claim that there was no longer any difference between the rightists and the neutralists. Furthermore, Souphanouvong added, any resolutions made in Paris would almost certainly be sabotaged by the real rightist power, General Phoumi Nosavan.

The squabbling continued; the start of the summit was postponed.

Among Prince Souvanna Phouma's papers, I have found a copy of a letter which he wrote to Prince Souphanouvong on September 7 while both were in Paris before the summit was convened. A portion of this letter, translated from the French, reveals, I believe, certain qualities of its author and his view of his own position as the leader of the neutralists:

In your letter [of September third] you have raised a question pertaining to the leadership of the rightist party. Now you know that my capacity as leader of the neutralist party gives me no more authority in the party of the right than I have authority in your own party. . . .

I wish to remind you that the rightist party has at last decided, in order to contribute toward a reduction of the tension and toward a solution of the Lao problem, to place its troops under the authority of the Minister of National Defense of the Government of National Union. A proposal to do likewise has also been made to you. It would be a serious error on your part to believe that through my position as Prime Minister and Minister of National Defense I have become, as a result of the rightists' decision, the leader of their party. The party of the right remains as it has been—one of the three principal factions of Laos.

Finally, I wish to call your attention to the following: I am and remain a neutralist. I am defending the interests and aspirations of all those who seek the happiness and prosperity of Laos in neutralism, independence, and sovereignty.

In this same letter, Prince Souvanna showed his anger at Souphanouvong's exploitation of the defection, under pressure, of some neutralist soldiers on the Plain of Jars to the Pathet Lao. Souvanna claimed that these soldiers had been induced to defect through devious and disloyal means, and he added: "I categorically reject calling them 'authentic neutralist forces.' "

Days went by, and Philip and I were faced with the problem of deciding whether the *pourparlers* among the princes and among their representatives on the lower echelons constituted a part of the summit or were merely preliminary discussions.

In Prince Souvanna Phouma's journals, which he faithfully kept throughout the years, I find this entry under September 19: "Eight P.M. Dinner at Laperouse with Campbell James, Stieglitz and Chadbourn. *Affaire des americains.*" That dinner is memorable to me for several reasons.

Campbell James was that very British American intelligence officer from Vientiane and the bar of the Constellation. He, unlike many of his colleagues, had always been supportive of Souvanna and liked to think of himself as a personal friend of the prince. He came to Paris as his agency's representative for the summit and in his perpetually extravagant fashion decided to host a small dinner party for his friend at the restaurant, which in those days merited three stars in the Michelin and was among the costliest in Paris. Philip and I were his only other guests.

We gathered that evening in one of the small, handsome, upstairs private rooms of Laperouse, rooms that at the turn of the century had been reserved for far more sensual purposes than diplomacy. The prince was at ease and knew full well he was with admirers. I felt we could approach him as one does a favorite professor—but surely not as a classmate. His dignity was inherent. Furthermore, after his various experiences with the Americans during the five previous years, if he had demonstrated a certain aloofness, or even suspicion, that would have been understandable—but he did not. And yet in his comments, he did not refrain from speaking of the past, of mentioning again how U.S. Central Intelligence had supported Phoumi Nosavan and bore a responsibility for the Battle of Vientiane. But he was entirely aware that, with the Kennedy administration and with Averell Harriman's role for that administration in Southeast Asia, the U.S. attitude and policy had drastically changed. He also understood that with new American elections and a new administration, our foreign policy might once more be altered.

Although the prince was exceptionally familiar with Vietnam and the Vietnamese—he was a graduate of a *lycée* in Hanoi—he had made certain throughout these years, even when we Americans were beginning to build up our military aid program for Saigon, to keep the Lao issue separate from the Vietnamese civil war. Both the little kingdom and South Vietnam were being attacked and invaded by the same enemy, North Vietnam, but Souvanna tried to make the world realize that the Lao cause was different—and unique.

At this Paris summit, Souvanna, I believe, thought that he could persuade his younger half-brother to bring the Pathet Lao back into the tripartite government as a permanent faction in accordance with the Geneva agreements. I think that Souvanna may have underestimated Souphanouvong's capacity to betray their cousin, the king. The two half-brothers were not unlike figures in a Shakespearean history. Our genial host and the waiters did not provide what might be called an unnoticed background for the conversation. I remember too many of the details. Before the meal our appetites were whetted by whiskey or champagne or both.

With the fish course, we drank a splendid white Montrachet, with the roast, the prince's favorite Cheval Blanc, with the raspberry souffle, a Château d'Yquem, and with the coffee and afterward, an ancient Napoleon brandy. Each wine was of a rare vintage, and once a bottle was uncorked, no drop was to be wasted.

The prince, a true epicure, enjoyed the repast without ever allowing the flow of wine to disrupt the discussion of Lao-American relations and the security and economic situation of the kingdom. Dinner and conversation lasted for hours.

The next afternoon I attended a wedding reception for a colleague at the embassy, and as I put a glass of champagne to my lips, a sensation I have rarely experienced seized me: my head started to spin. No, twirl. The previous evening's wines and brandy had their revenge. I made my way as inconspicuously as I could from the reception and got back to my flat and bed. I reeled from the ravages of diplomacy.

At last on the twenty-first day of September, the summit had its first official session at the château in Saint-Cloud. The three princes and the delegates from the three factions numbered in all some twelve negotiations plus a bevy of secretaries and assistants.

The three factions agreed that there were several major points to consider. The first, on which there was most accord, was to resolve national problems through pacific means and an immediate cease-fire. The second point dealt with conveying a new fourteen-nation conference on Laos, and here there were important disagreements, which centered on preconditions and the formation and control of the Lao delegation to such a conference. The third point at which they never arrived was whether the seat of the Government of National Union should remain in Vientiane, or be moved up to Luang Prabang, or as a major concession to the Pathet Lao be moved to their territory.

The princes remained at the summit for several days—some of the other delegates for several weeks—but then, sadly, another summit ended not with a resolution but with a lingering, indefinite negativism. And I resumed my work as field officer for France.

◆ ◆ ◆

Although this book attempts to relate the history of the last years of the little kingdom and depends not only upon memory but upon as much research as can be uncovered, I do not pretend to be a historian, which may unfortunately be all too evident. If I were one, I might ignore the incident I am about to recount, or I might find in it some significance that escaped this amateur. After these many years, I am still puzzled by it.

A month or so after the Paris conference had wound its way down, I received a message that General Phoumi Nosavan wished to see me the following morning at ten o'clock at the Lao embassy. I had heard that he was in Paris but could not imagine why he would send for me.

In proper bureaucratic fashion, and in this instance it made good sense, I called on the political officer of our embassy who looked after Asian affairs. He informed me that Phoumi was in Paris after a visit to Moscow. How strange—Phoumi Nosavan in Moscow! He had gained his fame, his wealth, and his position by proclaiming himself to be the most uncompromising of anti-communists. His Russian voyage seemed preposterous despite the complex maneuvering that went on in the endless struggle for power. Since Phoumi could not have gone there without the approval of the Soviet government, one wondered what their objective could have been. Surely they were not hoping to convert him. Or were they? Or had Phoumi requested the meeting in order to prove to the Soviets, who had always strongly opposed him, that they were wrong to do so for he was a closet anti-American? After all, the Americans had forsaken him to support the neutralists. Could an extreme right-winger suddenly align himself with the communists? There had been a notable precedent on the eve of World War II. But this was obviously wild speculation, and the political officer with whom I was speaking could offer no plausible reason why Phoumi had asked to see me.

The next morning at his residence, Ambassador Nouphat Chounramany greeted me briefly and deposited me in the salon. Soon the general entered. Phoumi had a tendency to put on weight, and that day he looked somewhat bloated and tired. He welcomed me austerely. A servant brought in coffee, and we sat and drank.

He told me he had been to Moscow, and I asked questions about his trip. His answers were equivocal. He had seen the Soviet Foreign Minister, but he was evasive as to what they had discussed.

He did state that he would soon be returning to Vientiane and expressed the hope that the situation there would improve. He suggested that his visit to Moscow might prove to be helpful.

That was all. There was nothing further. Nothing he had to discuss with me, no revelations, no material that merited even a lowly "restricted" on the diplomatic scale of confidentiality.

Then why had he sent for me? If it were merely to report his innocuous remarks back to the embassy and to Washington, why through a cultural affairs officer? He should have had as his diplomatic confidant one of the American political officers whose function it is to relay such messages.

Furthermore, ever since my days in Savannakhet when I was a sometime neighbor of his, the general may have been aware, I suspect, of my mistrust of him and his overriding ambitions. He may even have had an inkling of my decidedly pro-Souvanna sympathies.

Or was this precisely the reason that he used me as a messenger on this occasion?

I do not know. And that morning in Paris was the last time I ever saw Phoumi.

◆ ◆ ◆

The next January, it was now 1965, I was invited again to the Lao embassy for a reception being given by the ambassador. Having attended several previous receptions there, I was not surprised to find in the handsome double salon a few ambassadors, several ministers, some officials from the Quai d'Orsay, and twelve or so elegant Parisian ladies. The latter chatted, sipped their champagne, nibbled on the hors d'oeuvres, and seemed to believe that they were demonstrating moral support for the little kingdom by attending parties at the Lao embassy.

I proceeded through the expected routine. After an exchange of remarks with Ambassador Nouphat and his warm, friendly wife, I made my way around, exchanging bits of information with those I knew and introducing myself to several I did not know. Then, recognizing that voiceless stir which often occurs when someone special enters a crowded room, I looked toward the door where a young woman had made her appearance. The elegant ladies stopped their chatting to study her, and several of the men edged toward where she was being deferentially greeted by Nouphat.

She was, I assumed, in her late twenties. She was slim and of medium height. Her eyes were slightly almond-shaped and set well apart. Her nose was straight except for a small flare of the nostrils. Her lips were full and sensuous but not heavy. Her long black hair was pulled back into a chignon. Her costume was unmistakably haute couture: a dark dress with a subtle print, a small hat, gloves, and high-heeled shoes that supported extraordinarily beautiful legs. Her expression was dominating, unrelentingly so, and yet somehow managed to escape being disdainful.

I crossed to the Lao deputy chief of mission to ask who this young woman was.

"La Comtesse de G." he replied. I employ here the nineteenth-century fictional convention of using only a letter for the name of a certain titled family.

"But she's Asian, isn't she?" I asked.

He laughed. "She is Lao. She is Princess Moune, the daughter of Prince and Princess Souvanna Phouma."

This made me at once aware of the strong family resemblance she bore.

A while later, seeing that Nouphat was between conversations, I asked him to present me.

"Of course, dear friend," he said.

We had to wait until the princess was free. Then he introduced me and walked away.

Eager, overeager, to build some relationship based upon associations, I immediately mentioned that I had on occasion played bridge with her father and that I knew her mother and Panya. She accepted my credentials without any acknowledgement that she had ever heard of me. She probably had not.

Then I delved into a discussion of the Paris conference of the three princes. She displayed an intimate and carefully educated knowledge of the situation. She made it evident that in the political morass facing her country she was convinced that her father's path of neutrality was the only course that held any possibilities for the future of the kingdom. She did this while speaking a beautifully enunciated French and asserted her viewpoint positively but without arrogance.

She gave me her full attention. She did not play the cocktail reception game of looking over one's shoulder to see with whom she should next be conversing. However, our conversation did not last long. A Quai d'Orsay man was demanding her attention.

Princess Moune had not indicated any wish to continue our very brief acquaintanceship. I was sorry for that, for as I left the residence, my thoughts were largely about her. I had found her cool, actually aloof, but absolutely fascinating.

The thought penetrated that Moune was another of Prince Souvanna's children, and I laughed to think that she certainly needed no looking after.

❁ ❁ ❁

In the aftermath of the Siho-Kouprasith coup d'état, General Kouprasith Abhay assumed a very different air. He had experienced public humiliation, but Prince Souvanna Phouma, although extremely exigent in all that concerned himself and his family, often—perhaps too often—forgave his enemies. In this instance, Kouprasith was allowed to remain in charge of the military in the Vientiane area and was named by the prime minister to the newly formed army command. Kouprasith from this time on was a staunch and enthusiastic figure in the neutralist government and, I suspect, was pleased to separate himself from some of his former cohorts.

Phoumi Nosavan viewed Kouprasith's new prominence and independence as a threat to his own position. In his rise to power, Phoumi had brought Kouprasith along with him. Together they had fought the Battle of Vientiane and had won. When their military fortunes ebbed and they had to accept defeat at the conference tables of Geneva, they had resisted full participation in the tripartite government. They had maintained the right-wing army as their army rather than as part of the national army, and they regarded neutralist Kong Le with as much suspicion as they regarded the Pathet Lao. But after the 1964 coup, Phoumi would never again trust Kouprasith. And that he, Phoumi, was in danger of becoming an outsider on the ladder of power rankled him.

Phoumi, as usual, concocted new schemes. Instead of acting vindictively against Siho Lamphouthacoul for having bypassed him in his coup, Phoumi saw the opportunity to exploit the rift between Kouprasith and Siho. Under his aegis, Phoumi arranged for Siho to return to his former position as the head of the national police. Phoumi achieved several purposes by this appointment: Siho was again dependent upon him, the important police force was kept politically allied to him, and Kouprasith's influence in the area was lessened.

Siho seized the opportunity to regain power. Without question, he hoped that this would give him a way of finding some measure of revenge against Kouprasith Abhay, the man at whose hands he had suffered ever since the days when he had been a servant in the Abhay household.

What had been a more or less united right in the kingdom's political composition approached at the end of 1964 a sharp confrontation within its own ranks. The prime minister called a meeting of the army high command in mid-January of 1965 and demanded an end to the disputes and bickering among the rightists in the military. He insisted that the Royal Army be strengthened. He reminded his generals that the Pathet Lao were making new incursions and would profit from any weaknesses within the Royal Army. Soon after this meeting, the Ministry of Defense announced that important changes were to be made in the Lao army command, an announcement that created obvious consternation among certain rightists.

A few days later, at the military section of Wat Tay airport, a series of explosions destroyed ten army aircraft. These ten planes represented half of the army's fighter-bomber strength. A spokesman declared that the explosions had been caused by a short circuit, and his explanation was greeted by an overtly cynical reaction.

January 31 was a Sunday, and that evening Vientiane enjoyed its customary calm. The burnished reds and magentas of the sunset across the Mekong permeated then faded into the city. Journalists and intelligence agents exchanged information at the bar of the Constellation, glamorously gowned girls danced with the customers at the Vieng Ratry, downtown movie houses projected their fare of Thai and Indian films, and at the recreation room of the USAID compound the weekly duplicate bridge tournament was being played.

At half past eight, the calm was replaced by the arrival in trucks and jeeps and on foot of hundreds of armed soldiers. Their appearance made it all too clear that another coup was underway. Yes, the lightly guarded radio station was seized, and yes, the colonel in charge of the soldiers announced that the city was under his command. Kouprasith from his home at Camp Chinaimo sent out four of his soldiers to investigate. They were stopped at a roadblock, where two of them were killed by the blast of a machine gun manned by the rebels. The coup, however, completely failed to galvanize the city as a coup must do if it is to succeed, and by noon on Monday it seemed to have ended. But soon new rebel troops poured into the city from the provinces. Then it was discovered that the instigators of the coup were none other than that bumbling team of Phoumi and Siho.

It was high noon. It was Kouprasith versus Phoumi and Siho. The fighting quickly spread through the streets of the city. The national police under Siho fought with the rebels, while government troops were flown down from Luang Prabang to support the loyalists. Machine guns and tanks played their deadly roles. Shells were fired indiscriminately. Some sixty civilians were killed, and thousands more fled across the Mekong in *pirogues*.

By nightfall, a determined Kouprasith had defeated the rebels. Phoumi and Siho fled, with Kouprasith's men in hot pursuit, but the two generals managed to get to Thailand and a military base, where they placed themselves in the custody of the Thai army.

The Thai government and the Thai army had long treated Phoumi Nosavan as their favorite cousin and had supported him well beyond what the rules of national sovereignty permit. On this occasion, the Thais, a signatory nation to the Geneva accords, were embarrassed and could do no more for him than to offer him asylum.

The Lao government made the request, strongly endorsed by the United States and other governments, that the Thais not allow Phoumi the freedom to roam about, and especially not near the Lao border. The Thais acceded and installed him in a pleasant house in the southern town of Songkhla on the Gulf of Siam. I have visited Songkhla several times. It is an attractive town whose unspoiled beaches that stretch along intensely blue water make the site conducive—or even compulsive—to quiet reflection and therefore, I imagine, exactly what Phoumi did not want.

During the months that followed, at least four more attempts were made within the kingdom by Phoumi advocates to rebel against the government, but each such attempt was effectively stamped out by Kouprasith's soldiers. Phoumi and Siho's failed coup was the last true threat to the government from the right wing. After it, Prince Souvanna Phouma could for the first time depend upon a united army of rightists and neutralists. The Pathet Lao remained apart, unquestionably viewing this new rapprochement with regret.

Not having found the sanctuary in Thailand that was offered to Phoumi, Siho surprised almost everyone by reappearing in Vientiane in the summer of 1966. He claimed that he sought refuge from followers of Phoumi who were trying to murder him. He was placed in an army security prison, and some weeks later, so the explanation went, was "killed while trying to escape."

◆ ◆ ◆

I met the Count de G. He was an aristocratic-looking Frenchman but not otherwise impressive. It was at a reception, and he was there with Princess Moune. She was friendly, introduced me to him, and revealed in her remarks that she was better informed about me now than she had been. I was pleased to think that perhaps she had made inquiries about me. On this occasion she was if anything even more extraordinary in appearance, for she was wearing a traditional Lao costume, the dark blue silk skirt embroidered in heavy silver, a blue shirt, and a scarf of the same dark blue and silver worn across one shoulder. I had to be careful. I wanted to spend the remainder of the evening speaking only with her, which of course is not acceptable at a diplomatic reception.

I met his mother, the Countess de G. She was Swiss rather than French, a widow, and the proprietress of a finishing school in Florence to which some of the most affluent American families sent their daughters. An aggressive woman, she decided that since I was a friend of her son-in-law and was in the cultural affairs section of the American embassy, I might prove helpful to her school. Accordingly, she several times called on me at my office.

In July, Prince Souvanna Phouma came to Paris. He was making official visits to several heads of state, including General de

Gaulle, and so spent days in France. He and the princess had a few friends to their apartment one evening, and I had the opportunity of a brief conversation with him. He was preparing for national elections in September and was splendidly confident that he was doing for the little kingdom whatever could be done to expand its democracy and guard its neutrality. I always found it to be a rare experience when in his presence.

My constant travels about France kept me away from Paris, and I had only one other occasion that year to see the young count and his princess, but as winter approached, his mother invited me to spend the Christmas holiday period at her school in Italy. There would be no students present, only invited friends. For several reasons, I was unable to accept her generous invitation, but if I had, I might have celebrated the end of the year with Moune.

❁ ❁ ❁

Phoumi Nosavan's abrupt departure left open the leadership of the kingdom's rightist faction. The nominal head of the right, Prince Boun Oum, was at once called upon to replace Phoumi as deputy prime minister, but the prince did not have his heart in it. He preferred to spend his time in his own fiefdom of Champassak when he was not in Paris or on the French Riviera. He had never cared for Vientiane.

Members of the mandarin Sananikone family were eager to fill the gap. There was the jovial but ambitious Ngon, who held a ministerial post in the cabinet, his somewhat dissipated brother Oune, who was a general in the army, and elder brother Phoui, who as head of the National Assembly tried to make matters difficult for his arch rival, Prince Souvanna. But none of the Sananikones succeeded in assuming the authority of the deposed leader. As for Kouprasith Abhay, who was related to the Sananikones, he remained exclusively a military force.

New elections for the National Assembly were held in September of 1965. They were being held because this tiny, developing monarchy in a constant state of crisis—with strong internal dissension and an ongoing invasion from its powerful, bellicose neighbor—refused to forgo a democratic basis and continued to hold elections for parliament whenever circumstances required. Furthermore, under Prince Souvanna Phouma these elections were honest, not rigged, and King Savang Vatthana, who often disagreed with his prime minister on many issues, upheld him in this matter. Equally extraordinary is that in each election the government's mortal enemy, the Pathet Lao was urged to participate.

The surprise of the September balloting was the success of the new Young People's party, which placed ten of its sixteen candidates in the National Assembly. The party was under the leadership of the recently appointed minister of finance, Sisouk na Champassak.

Sisouk was a nephew of Prince Boun Oum but was utterly unlike his uncle.

Educated largely in France, a graduate of the Institute of Political Science in Paris, he was handsome, charming, athletic, and remarkably intelligent. What is more, he had a passion for politics. An early venture in government had been unfortunate, for he was one of Phoumi's short-lived Defense Committee for the National Interest and had accordingly been ousted from the cabinet when the Prime Minister Phoui Sananikone could no longer tolerate the group's arrogance. But at the Geneva conference, Sisouk had been outstanding as a delegate for the rightists. He was then appointed Lao Ambassador to the United Nations, where he was a highly effective envoy, and managed while at that post to write a book, *Storm Over Laos*, which received much deserved attention. In 1965, Prince Souvanna appointed the thirty-seven-year-old Sisouk to be his minister of finance, and Sisouk in that role proved as incorruptible as the previous minister of finance, Phoumi Nosavan, had been unscrupulous.

During the next ten years, Sisouk became second only to Prince Souvanna as a leader of the Lao.

It should also be noted that the new American ambassador to Vientiane was William Healy Sullivan, an old friend of Sisouk. Bill Sullivan had served as Averell Harriman's deputy at the Geneva conference, and his friendship with Sisouk stemmed from days and evenings spent in discussion and argument on the shores of Lac Leman.

By 1965, Bill Sullivan had become a well-known State Department officer. He was a brilliant, extremely energetic, and most articulate diplomat. His was a feisty personality, but he was a loyal and valuable friend of the little kingdom.

How fortuitous it was that the great talents of Souvanna, Sisouk, and Sullivan were gathered there in this period to give Laos the inner political strength it absolutely needed.

❊ ❊ ❊

When the United States became preoccupied by and anguished over the war in South Vietnam, many unfairly assumed that what was happening in Laos was nothing but another aspect of that war. True, the little kingdom had a frontier in common with South Vietnam, and North Vietnam was the mutual enemy of both countries, but their situations were utterly different.

I maintain this although my statement may be more difficult to propound in regard to the events of 1965, when a certain important linkage occurred.

One of the most salient accords of the Geneva conference was that all foreign troops were to leave Laos. The North Vietnamese, signatory to the agreements, never observed them. The British government that year released a report which offered incontrovertible evidence that thousands of North Vietnamese soldiers were still present in Laos. The report had been written by the Indian and Canadian members of the International Control Commission. The Polish delegates to the commission had refused to participate in the investigation, and the Soviet government objected to the release of the report by the British.

Prince Souvanna Phouma and his neutralist government were painfully aware that the basis for the peace and independence of the kingdom was being consistently violated by the North Vietnamese. The Lao rightists taunted the prime minister with his ineffectiveness against the invaders, and Souvanna's hopes to bring his half-brother, Prince Souphanouvong, into a more conciliatory position were fading. As prime minister, Souvanna realized that since negotiations with the Pathet Lao did not progress, some drastic action had to be taken. Washington faced it own dilemma vis-à-vis the situation. The North Vietnamese regularly sent through the little kingdom vitally needed supplies for their soldiers in South Vietnam, a blatant exploitation of the Geneva accords. American troops were fighting in South Vietnam, but American soldiers had left Laos in accordance with the Geneva demands. This afforded to the North Vietnamese an overwhelming advantage.

At this point, the American and Lao governments decided on a course of action that was well analyzed by the Australian journalist Dennis Warner for the *Reporter* magazine of April 22, 1965:

> The United States had two choices: it could denounce the Geneva Agreements, openly intervene in the war once again, and perhaps lose the support of Souvanna and King Savang Vatthana; or it could follow the Pathet Lao ground rules. It chose the latter, and now from its own privileged sanctuaries in northeastern and northern Thailand, as well as from South Vietnam and the Seventh Fleet, it is working with the full approval of the Royal Lao government in an attempt to restore the balance destroyed by North Vietnam's disregard of the Geneva Agreements.

Prince Souvanna Phouma's approval of the plan for the bombing by aircraft, Lao and American, of the North Vietnamese invaders did not mean that Laos had entered the war as an ally of the United States. It did mean that if at that time the United States for reasons of its own was willing to help the little kingdom rid itself of the North Vietnamese incursions, Laos was going to accept such assistance.

The North Vietnamese, however, were not deterred, and by the end of the year there was increased talk of the Americans implementing their efforts by sending soldiers into Laos and perhaps Cambodia as well.

The Associated Press questioned Souvanna on this and other matters in a letter in late December, to which the prince responded in part by writing:

> First of all, Laos is an independent state. According to the 1962 agreements, its neutrality is guaranteed by thirteen nations, including the United States. Under the conditions and because of contracted obligations, there can be no question of the Government's accepting American troops in Laos to control the Ho Chi Minh Trail.
>
> The Geneva agreements would have no more being and the war in Laos would extend and become more intense. As for the international implications of such a violation of the Geneva accords, they are so dangerous that as long as I am chief of government, I will not involve my country in this adventure.

There were those in the American military command in Saigon who were unhappy with the prince's forthright statement and independence, and we shall hear from them later.

◆ ◆ ◆

My assignment in France kept me spinning, but pleasurably. I did my own planning and arranged American programs in such cities as Dijon, Bordeaux, Nantes, Avignon. Each program was cosponsored by municipal and university authorities, and each included exhibitions, concerts, and lecturers. Arthur Rubinstein and Isaac Stern were among those who performed for us. One exhibition was the first Pop Art show to tour the museums of the provinces. It included major paintings by Dine, Johns, Lichtenstein, Rauschenberg, Rosenquist, Warhol, and Wesselman and managed to distress most of the directors of the museums in which it was installed.

My travel schedule did allow me to be in Paris on the April date in 1966 I had been invited by Princess Souvanna Phouma to a party in her apartment in Auteuil. Upon arriving, I learned that the gathering was to celebrate Moune's birthday. Present were several friends as well as some colleagues from UNESCO, where Moune was serving on the Lao staff, but the Count de G. was conspicuously absent. In my conversations with the young princess, I was aware of a mind that was exceptionally keen and guileless. But she had, I thought, a troubled air. She did not smile nearly so often as I would have liked.

The next day I invented a reason to telephone Ambassador Nouphat at the Lao embassy. Planted in my conversation with him, posed as casually as I could muster, was a question about Princess Moune and the Count de G. Nouphat laughed, surprised that I did not know Moune was separated from her husband. He went on to say that he believed she was in the process of obtaining a divorce.

When I hung up the receiver, I sat at my desk with mixed emotions. I was unhappy for Moune's sake but unable to conceal my selfish elation. She was not yet legally single, but she was as of now socially unengaged, and her new status, I realized, concerned me enormously. Although I could not know it then, this was a landmark event in my life, as important for me, let us say, as the ultimate departure of Phoumi Nosavan was for the little kingdom.

Long reflection made me somewhat nervous. My relationship with Princess Moune was very slight and, far worse, not at all on the track that ordinarily a man might take in approaching an eligible woman. To begin with, I was in awe of her father. Then, to my embarrassment, I had to admit I was a bit in awe of her. Therefore, I could not anticipate a romantic escapade—and certainly not a permanent alliance with the formidable princess. But simply to learn that she was now free raised my pulse rate.

At once I started planning or plotting various ways to spend time with her. It would be imprudent, I felt, to rush things, but told myself that since I was capable of inventing programs throughout France, I should be able to invent ways of getting to see her. Subtlety was required. I could not simply telephone to ask, "What are you doing this evening, *Altesse*?" Perhaps I should have tried that direct method, but I lacked the chutzpa.

My campaign proceeded. She accompanied me to a *vernissage*, and I noted that she readily distinguished bad art from good—or should I say, we saw eye to eye about painting. We went to the theater—she was a severe, perceptive, but appreciative critic. She was my guest at a large reception at the American ambassador's residence and was naturally both skillful and at ease in addressing the attention she received at a large diplomatic reception. Gabrielle, my good Burgundian woman, was forever urging me to entertain at my apartment—she wanted the guests to admire her cooking—and so I found reasons, a visitor or an event, to have a series of small cocktail and dinner parties. To some Moune came, and to some she did not, although she was invited to all of them. Once in a while we went out for dinner, just the two of us. She invited me to her attractive apartment for dinner and bridge with French friends. Her bridge game was not on the level of her father's—few are on that level—but she played an astute game. I pressed my luck further when spending time in Toulouse for the *Mois Américain* I had organized. A performance of *Porgy and Bess* at the local opera house became the excuse for telephoning Paris to invite her to Toulouse for the weekend. She sounded amused at the invitation, but declined.

We were having dinner at one of my favorite small Paris restaurants. She, as always, looked marvelous and elegant. She wore, I recall, a black suit with a fur collar and large gold earrings, which I recognized as Laotian. I asked if the heavy gold bracelet she wore also came from there. No, she replied offhandedly, it was a gift from Prince Sihanouk.

We talked about recent developments in the kingdom and then there was a pause—a prolonged pause. Her limpid eyes peered into mine and she said matter-of-factly: "I'm returning to Laos next month."

"For a visit?" I demanded, hoping for an affirmation.

No, she explained, she was going to work at the Ministry of Foreign Affairs. Her position had already been designated. She would be *chef de cabinet*, an important function at the Ministry.

This news was reasonable. Her background and her education had been careful preparation for a career in international affairs on behalf of her country. It made perfect sense. With her marriage to a Frenchman about to be dissolved, and with her position at UNESCO insufficiently demanding, there was no urgent reason for her to remain in Paris while there were good reasons for her to return home.

I should have expected this development but had not allowed myself to think about it. This was vexing. She was leaving and what we had was something akin to friendship—not at all what I had wanted it to be. But I also realized that I had made no serious effort to change the nature of our relationship because such an effort might have destroyed it and left me with no relationship at all with Moune. Now I regretted my forbearance, but it was too late.

While I was on one of my trips to the provinces, Moune took her departure from France.

❋ ❋ ❋

The Lao National Assembly continued to be dominated by the rightists, who rejected the fiscal policies proffered to them by Prime Minister Prince Souvanna Phouma in October 1966. Consequently the Assembly was disbanded and new elections were scheduled. These were held on the first day of 1967, and some eight hundred thousand persons were declared eligible to vote. These included many who were illiterate but who could identify the candidates of their choice at the voting polls—generally located at the pagodas or schools.

And so the little kingdom, under strongly adverse circumstances, held another free and non violent election. There were one hundred and forty one candidates, from which fifty-nine members of the new Assembly were chosen. As he had consistently done in the past, Prince Souvanna Phouma urged the Pathet Lao to take part in the balloting, and they refused. The tripartite neutralist government was upheld by the voters, and the National Assembly was once more headed by the rightist Phoui Sananikone.

The Pathet Lao kept a low profile, unquestionably because their mentors, the North Vietnamese, were too involved in their broadening war in South Vietnam, where they were fighting American soldiers. Nevertheless, Prince Souvanna, who declared himself pleased with the results, announced that the four cabinet posts reserved for the Pathet Lao were being kept open for them.

Oh little kingdom, how utterly exceptional you and your prime minister were!

◆ ◆ ◆

A personnel officer from Washington came into my office at the embassy one afternoon in June 1967. His visit was not casual; he was there with a mission. An unsympathetic, bureaucratic type, he displayed not one iota of concern for those whose assignments—and therefore destinies—he was tampering with, but rather was exclusively bent on filling the agency's demands for a sufficient number of live bodies in Saigon. It was a though the agency believed that if it got enough of us there, we could not all be eradicated. He emphasized that with my Southeast Asia background I was a natural for this posting and should prepare myself to move on to Vietnam.

That prospect held no attraction for me. Furthermore, with Moune back in Laos, I wanted to go back to Laos.

I rose to the occasion and made out a splendid case for Vientiane as my next post: I knew the kingdom well; I had been and would be an effective officer there; I had some familiarity with the language; and finally, I was asking for an assignment that few people ever requested.

The personnel man heard my arguments and left. The next day he came back to the office, visibly resentful to bring me excellent tidings. He had been on the phone with Washington and learned that the cultural attaché position at the Vientiane embassy would be open in November. He informed Washington of my request.

A few weeks later, a cable from Washington announced that I was indeed to be the new cultural attaché in Laos.

◆ ◆ ◆

Au revoir, Paris, and back to the United States for home leave. Up and down the East Coast I visited friends and museums, attended concerts and the theater, and as is my preference, danced in night clubs rather than watched ballets.

My Washington briefing was scheduled for late October. What is dubiously called a briefing means stopping by at the various

Photographs

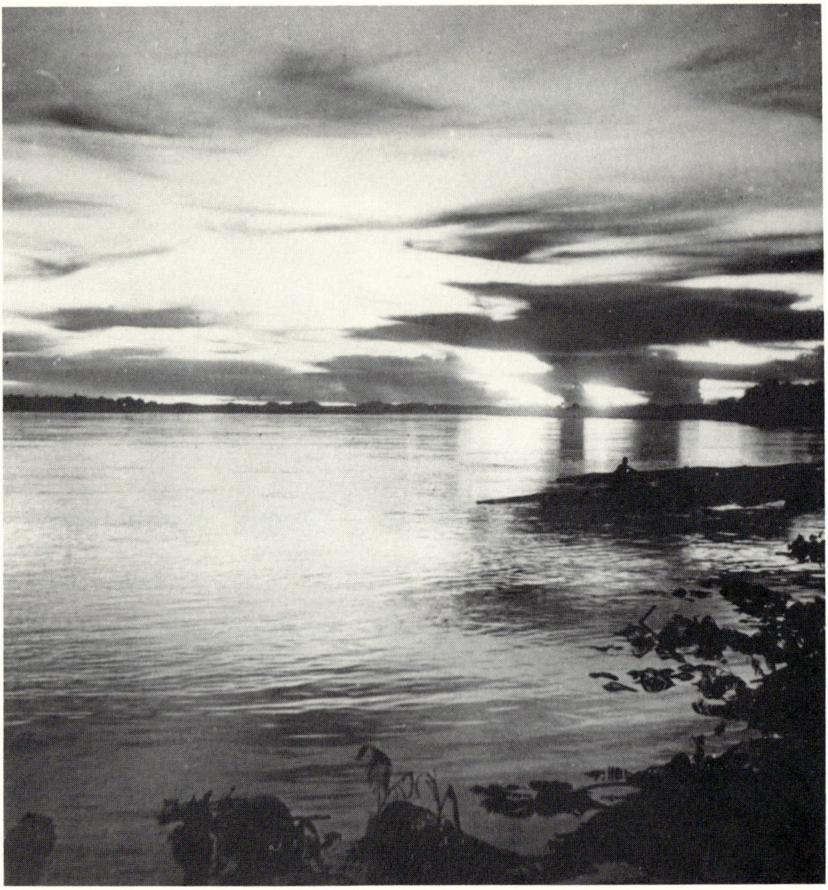

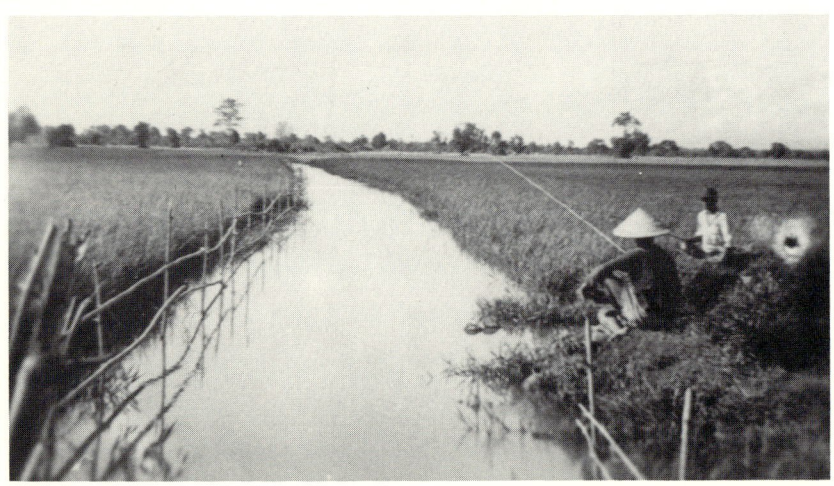

Sunset on the Mekong river.

A rice paddy outside Vientiane.

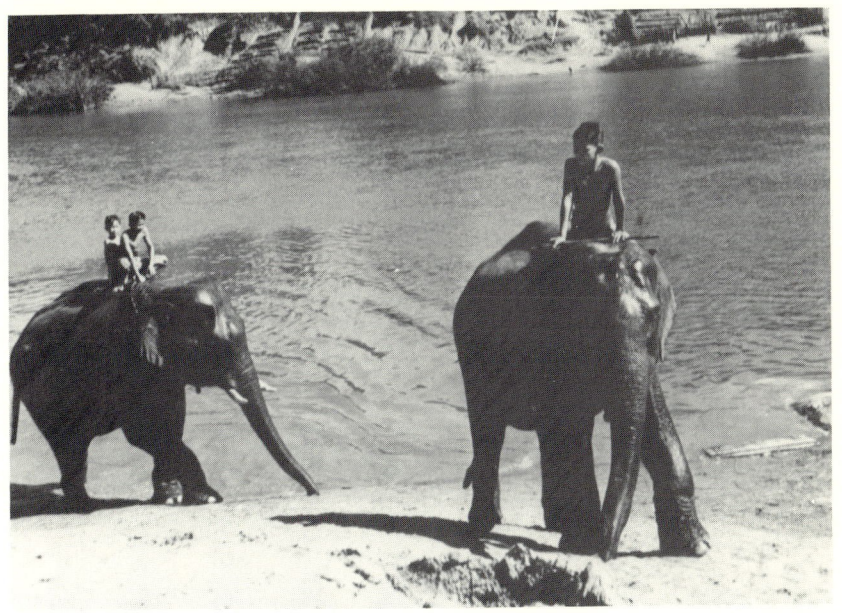

Lao children and elephants.

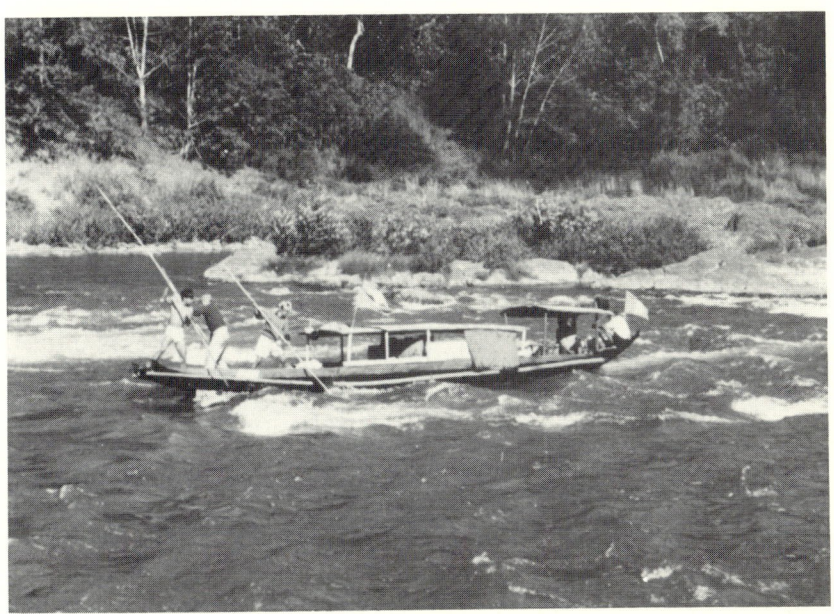

A *pirogue* fighting rapids on the Mekong river.

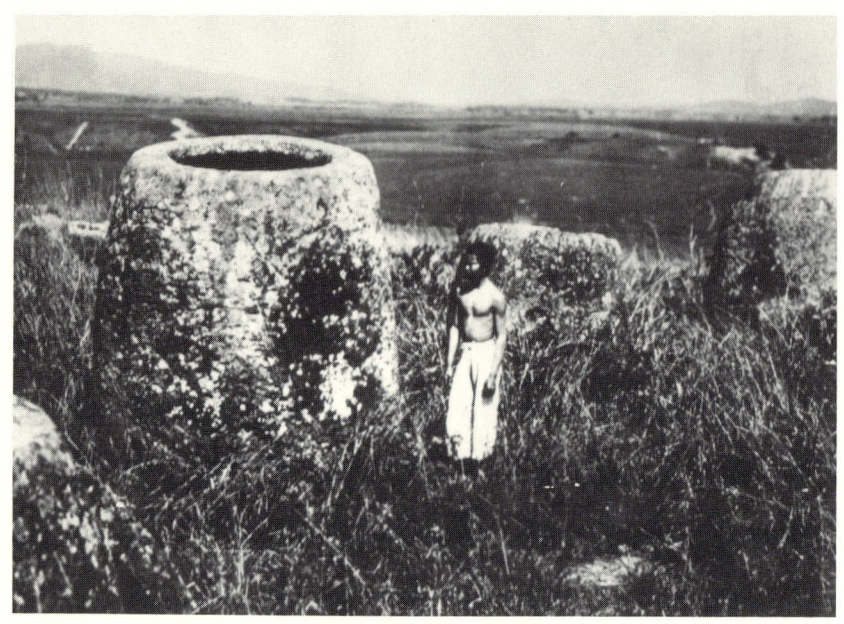

The Plain of Jars.

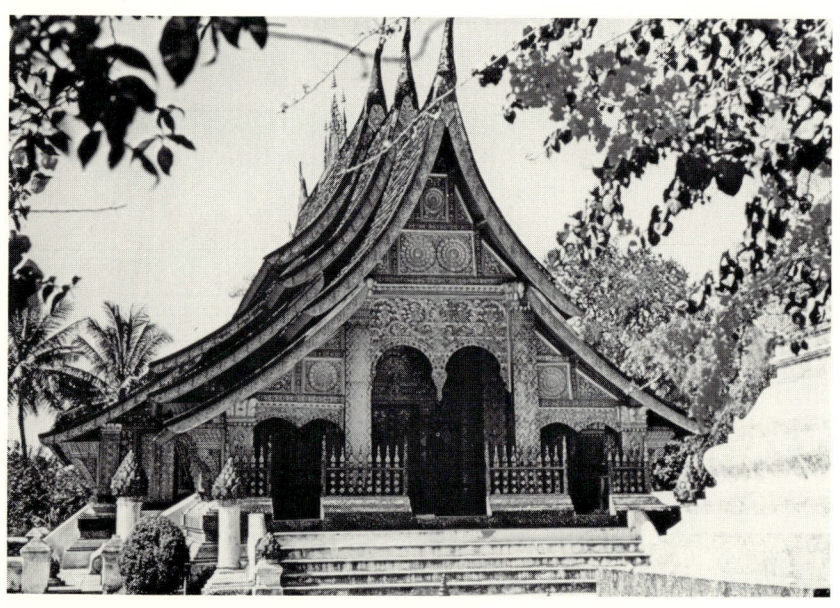

Vat Sieng Mouane, a temple in Luang Prabang.

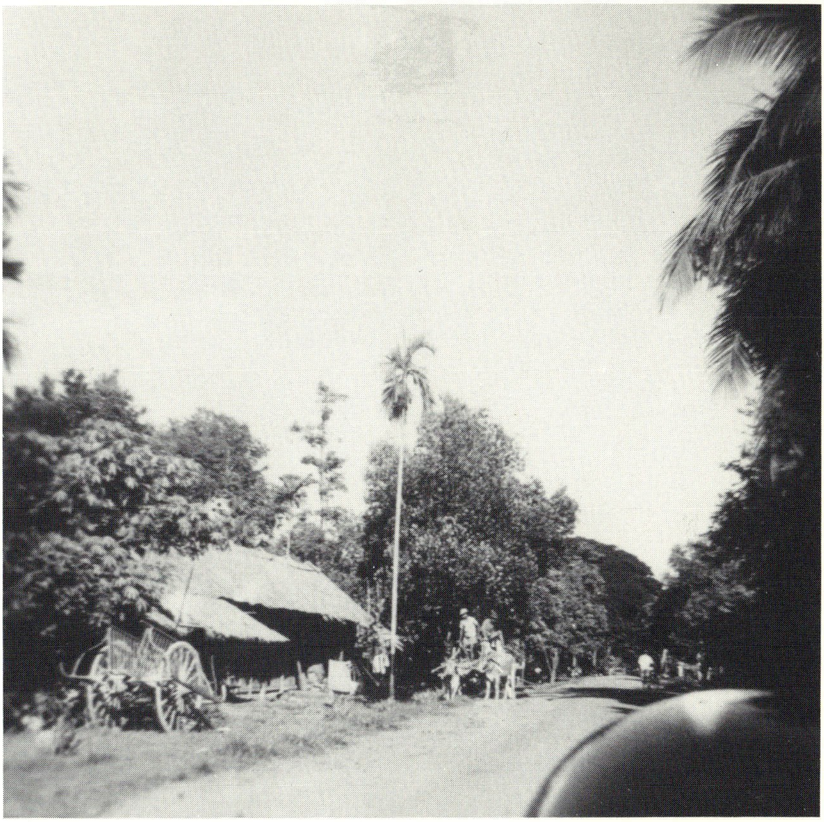

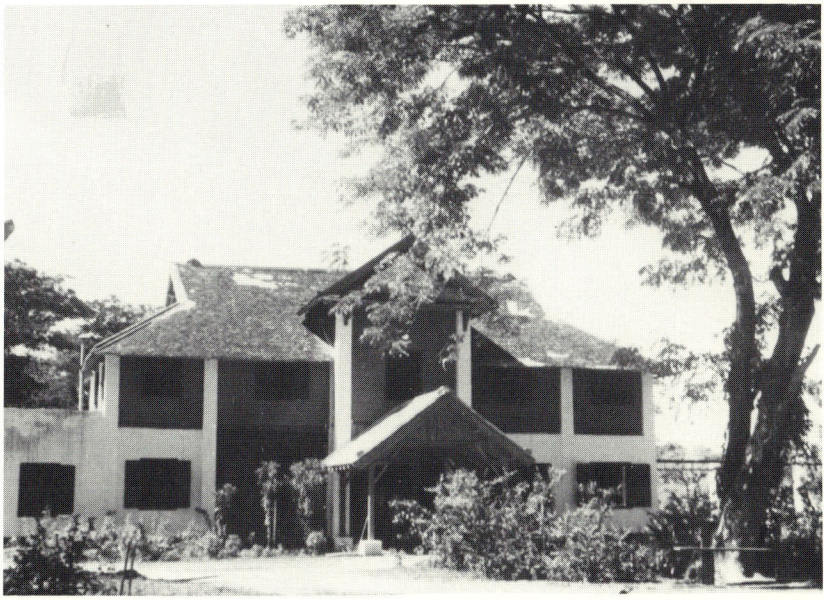

A Lao village between Vientiane and Nong Thevada.

Prince and Princess Souvanna Phouma's country home, Nong Thevada.

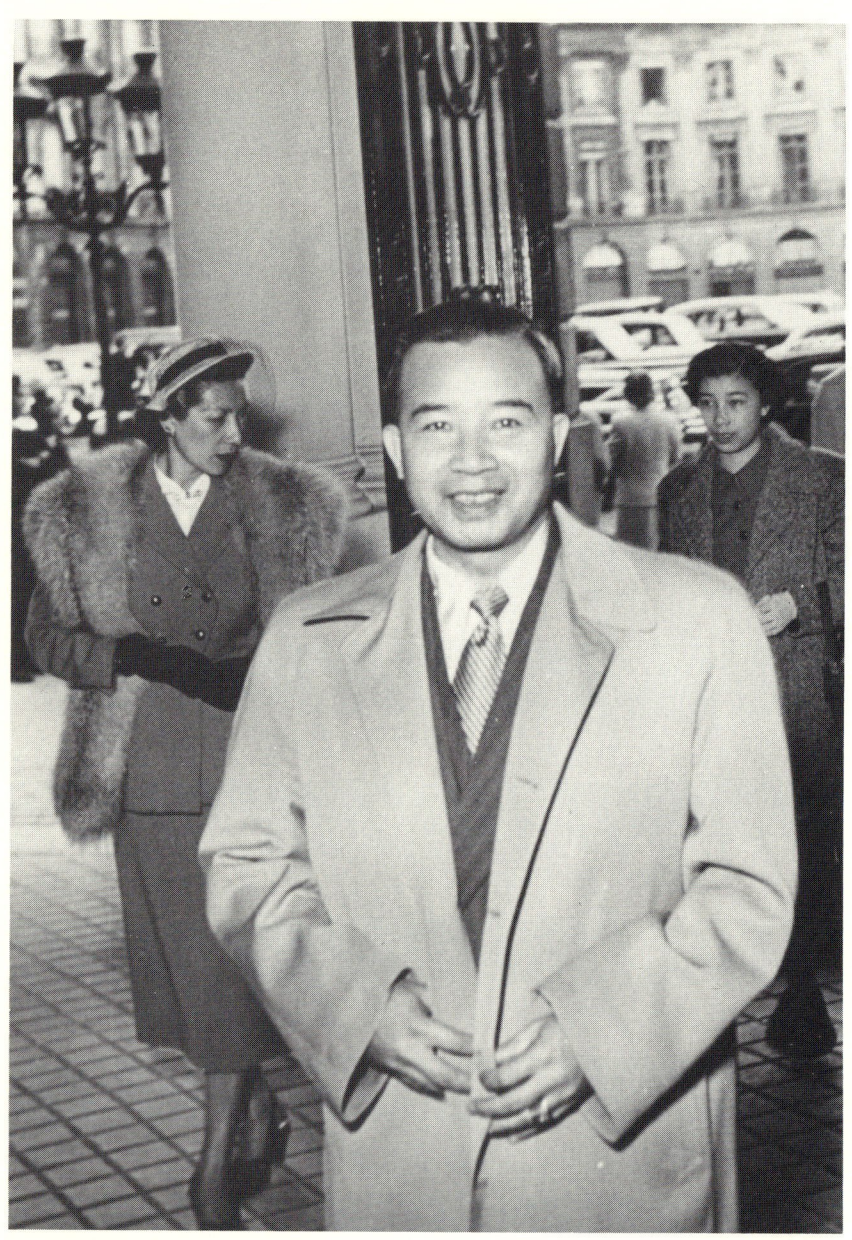

Prince and Princess Souvanna Phouma accompanied by their daughter Princess Moune, Paris 1952.

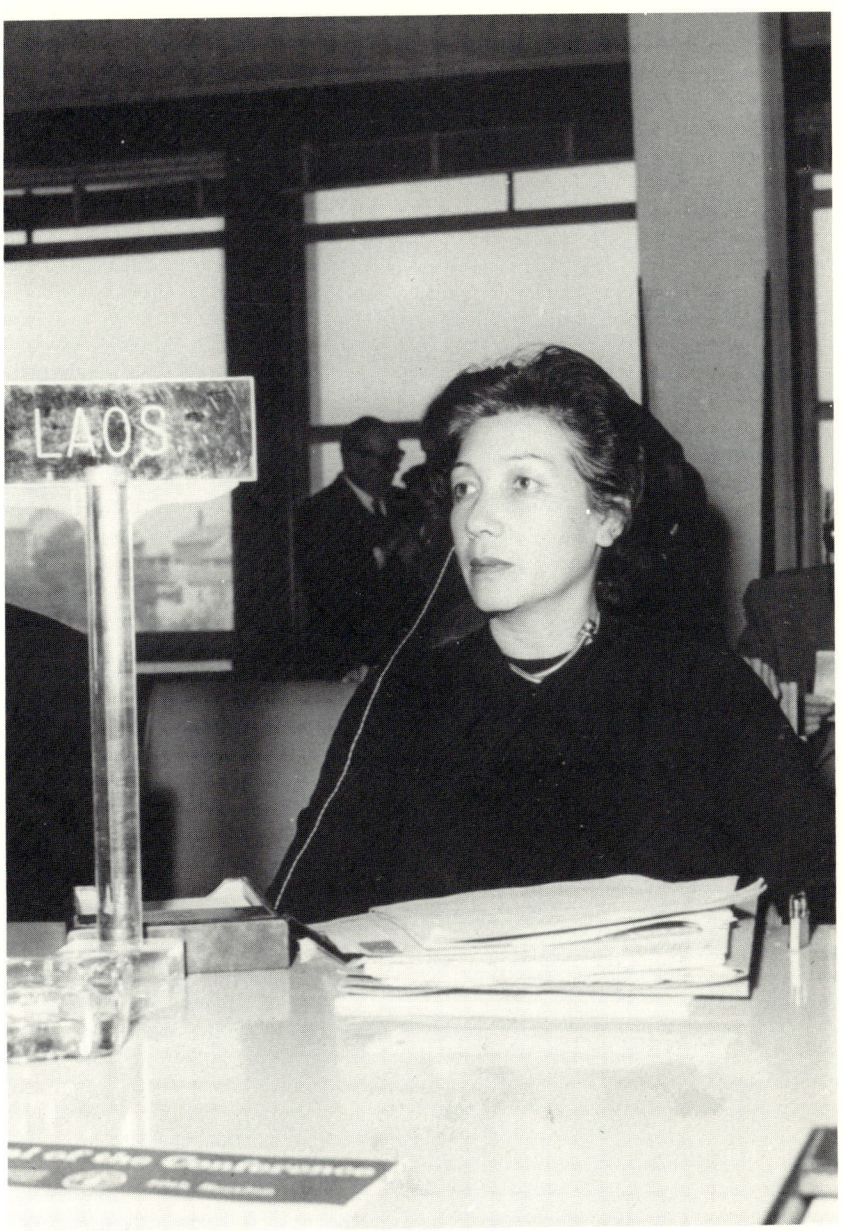

Princess Souvanna Phouma representing Laos at a F.A.O. conference.

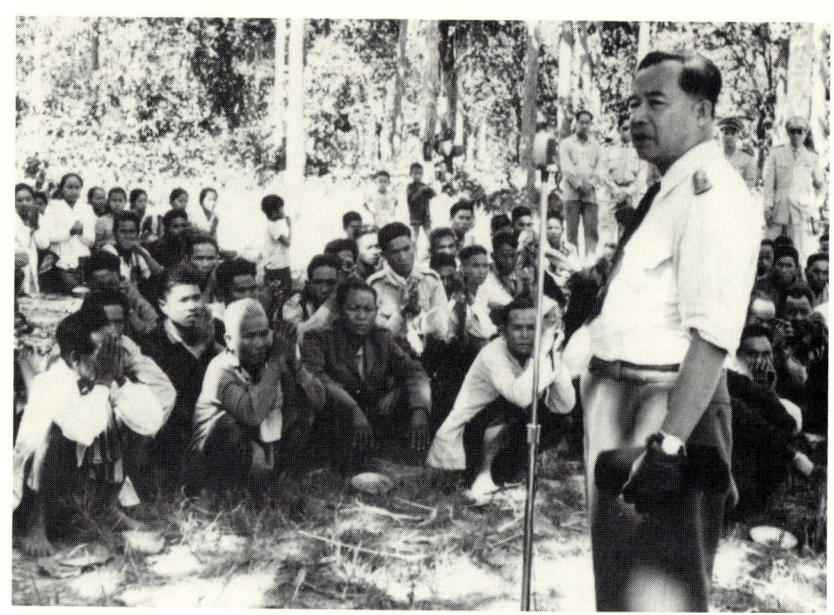

Prince Souvanna Phouma addressing villagers in northern Laos.

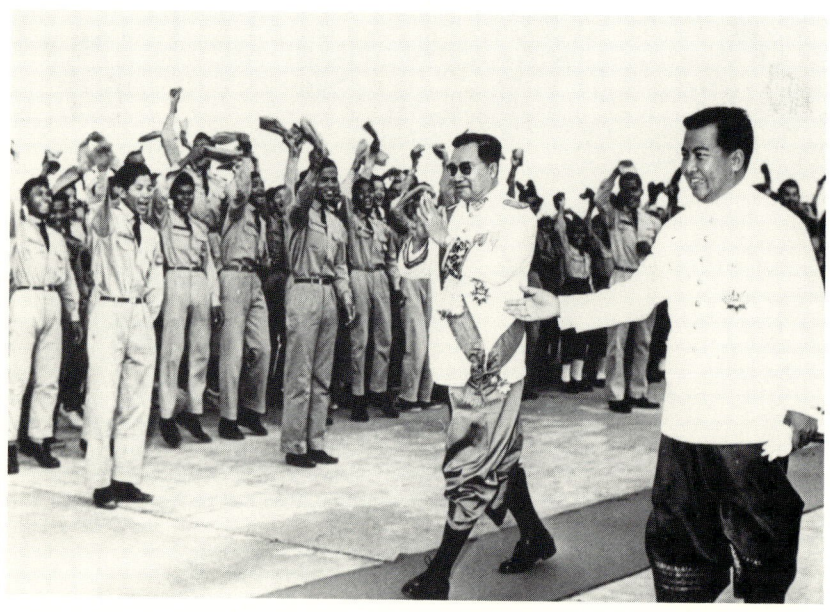

Prince Sihanouk receiving Prince Souvanna Phouma in Phnom Penh.

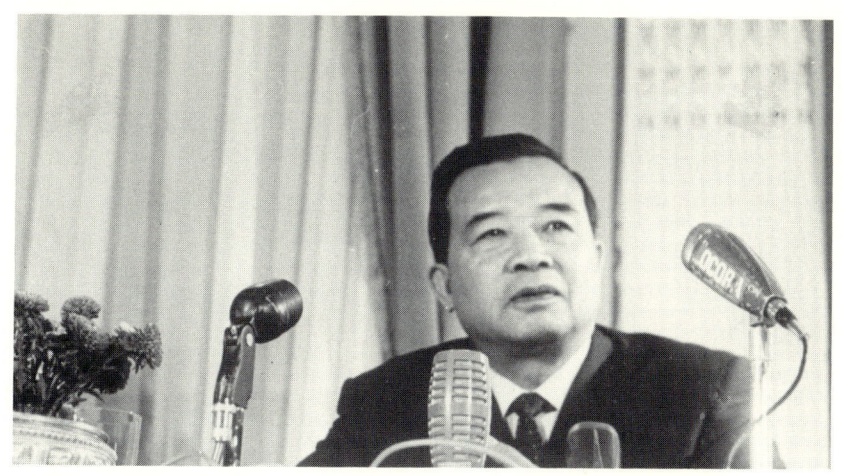

Prince Souvanna Phouma giving a press conference.

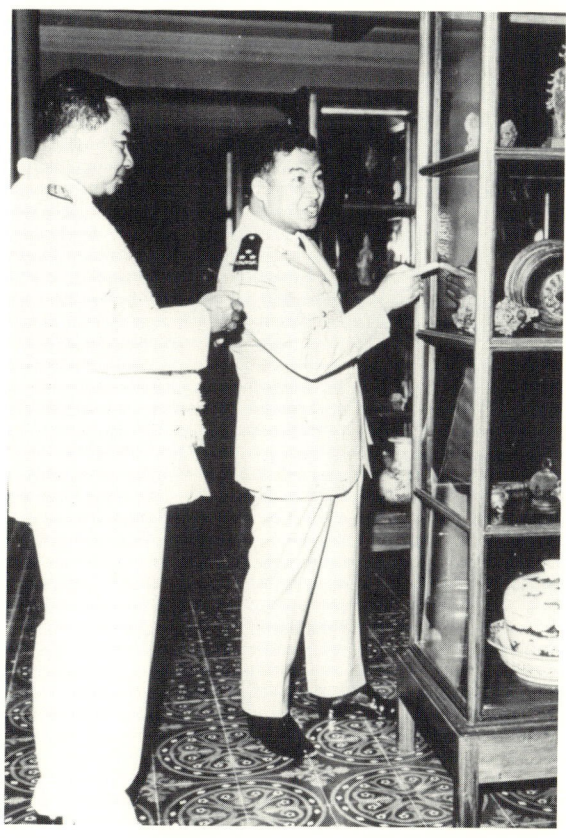

HRH Prince Norodom Sihanouk and Prince Souvanna Phouma
at the Royal Palace Museum, Phnom Penh.

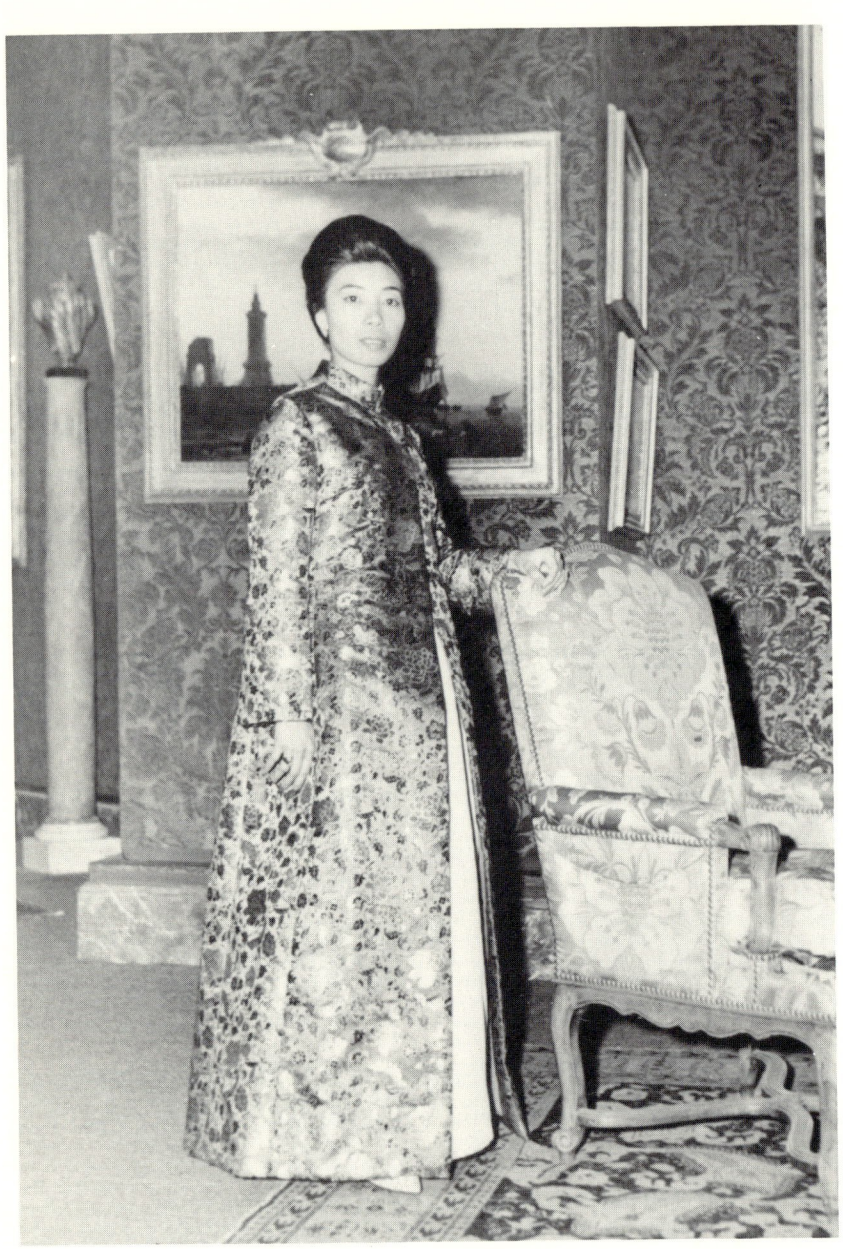

Princess Moune, Paris 1964.

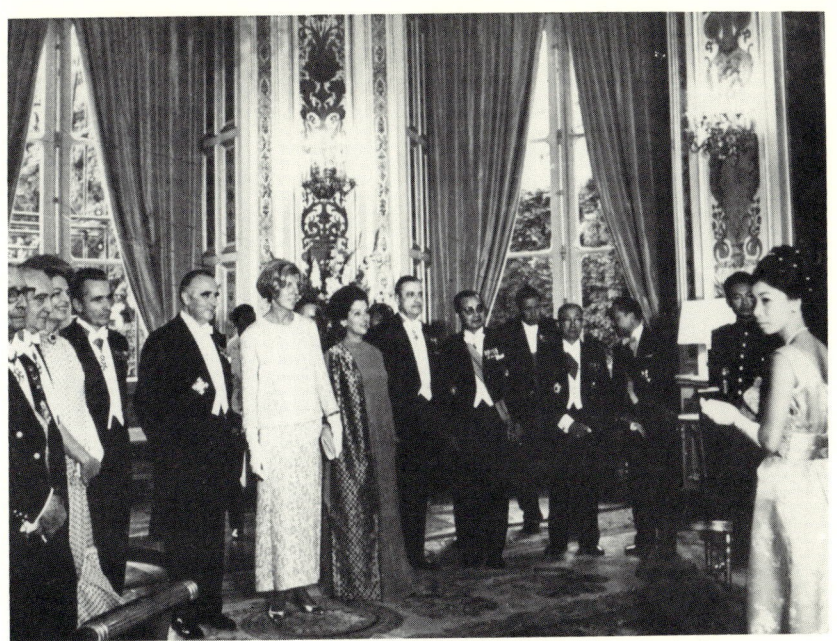

Prime Minister Souvanna Phouma and Lao dignitaries with Prime Minister and Mme. Pompidou at the Elysée palace.

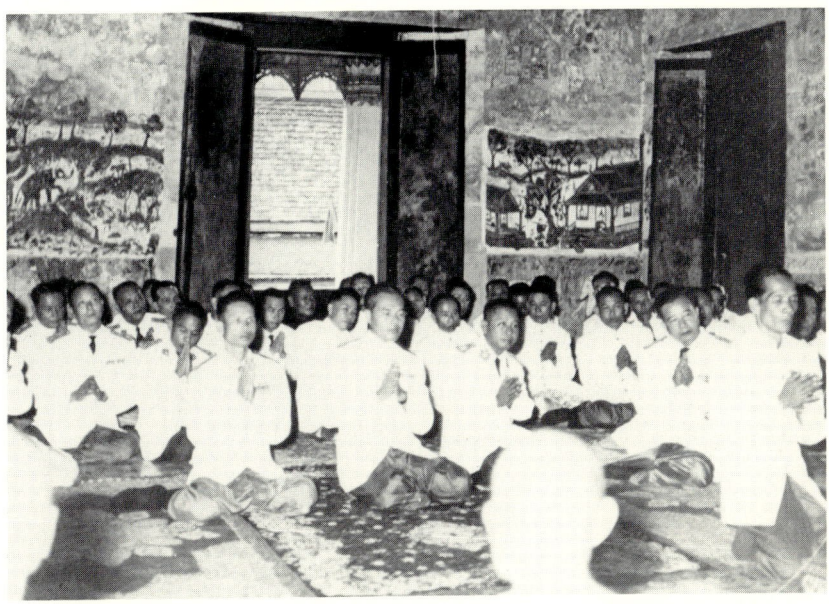

Members of the government attending a religious ceremony at the pagoda, Vientiane.

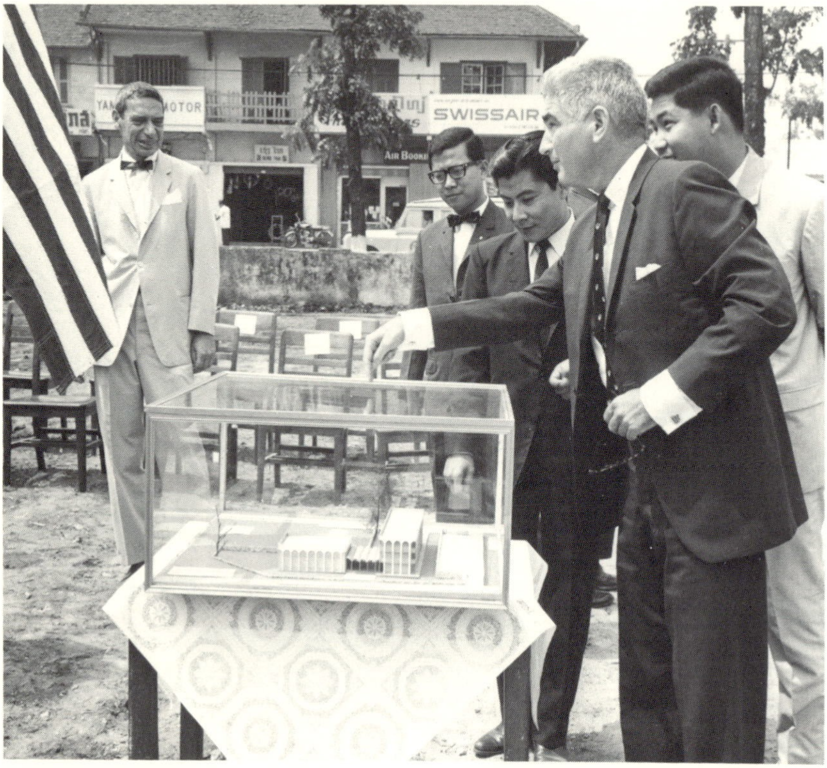

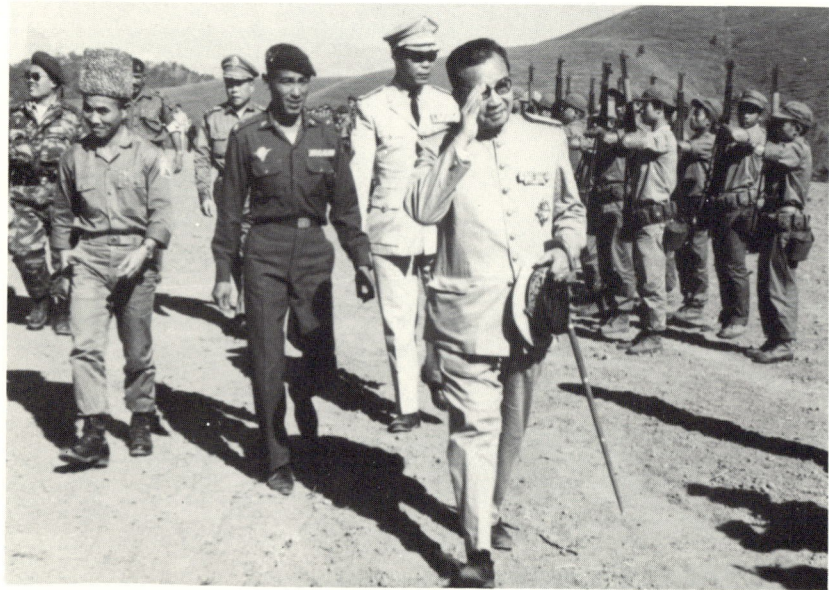

American Ambassador William H. Sullivan, Cultural Attaché Perry J. Stieglitz, and Lao board members inspecting model of the New Lao-American Association.

Prince Souvanna Phouma reviewing neutralist troops in Northern Laos, with Captain Kong Le (in the fur hat, far left) 1964.

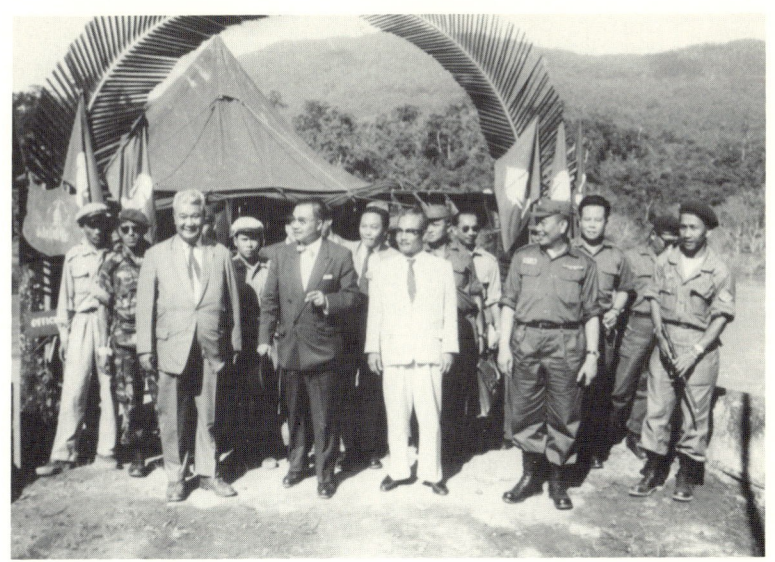

The "Three Princes" meeting at Hin Heup (October 1961). Front row from left to right: Prince Boun Oum, Prince Souvanna Phouma, Prince Souphanouvong (in white), and General Phoumi Nosavan.

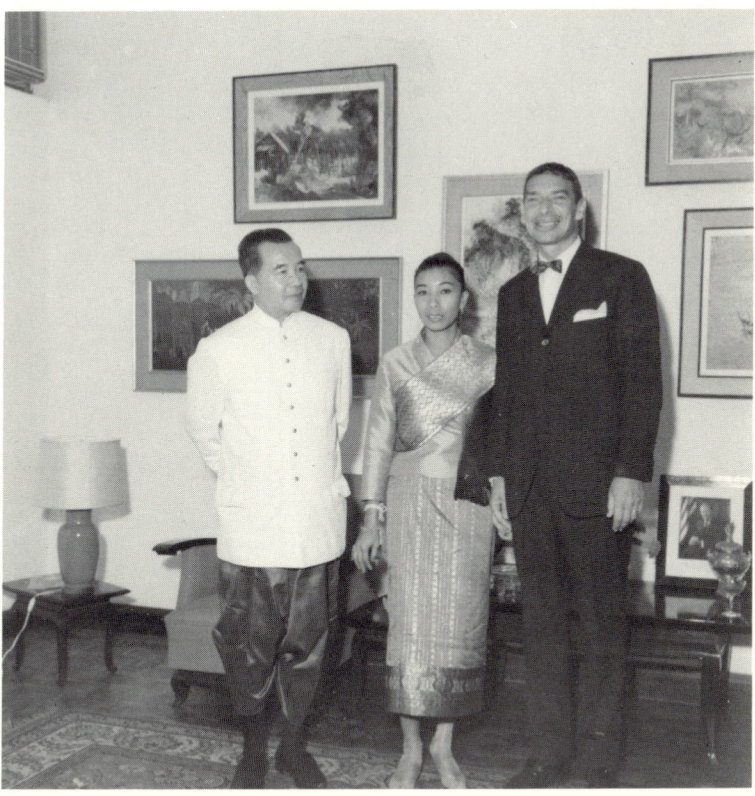

The wedding ceremony: Prince Souvanna Phouma and the newlyweds.

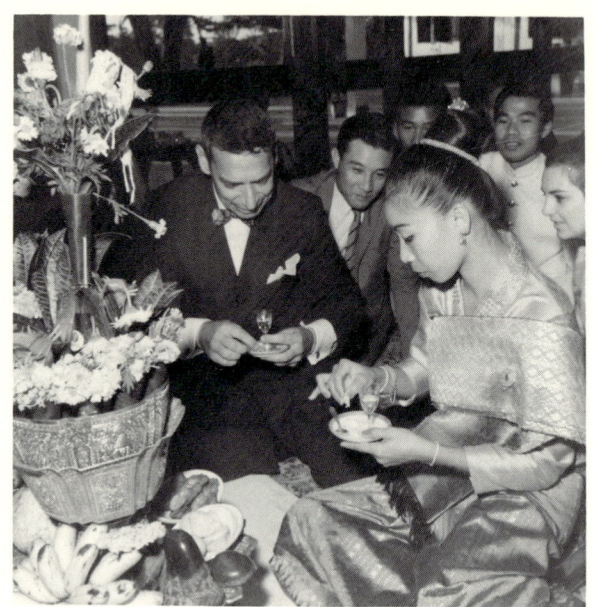

The wedding ceremony.

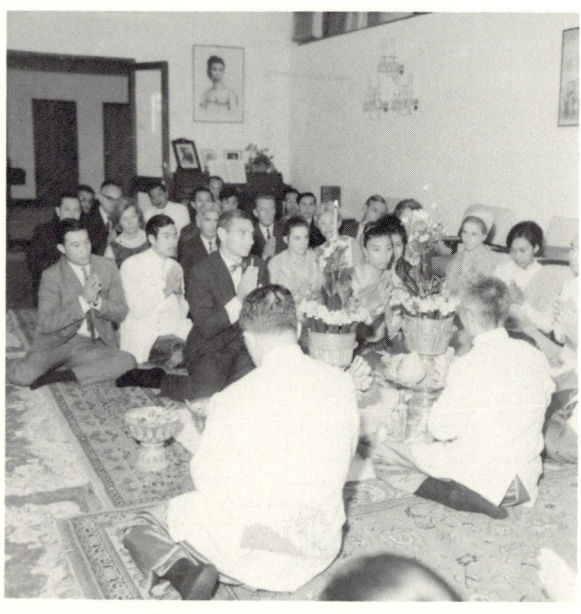

The wedding ceremony.

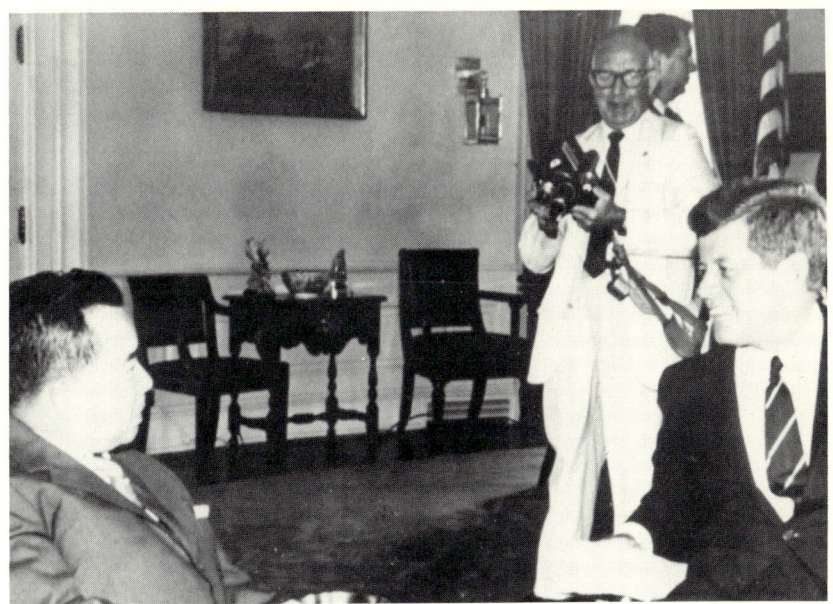

Prince Souvanna Phouma received by President Kennedy at the
White House.

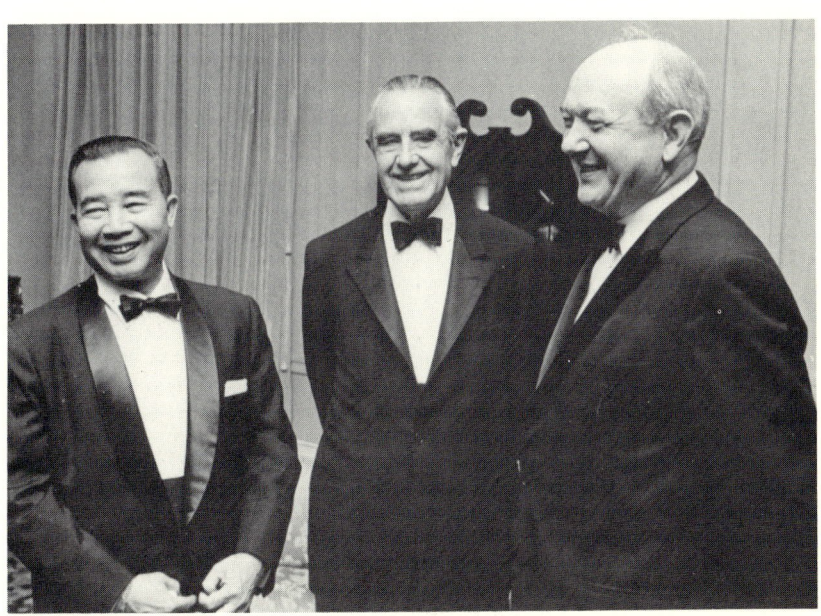

Prince Souvanna Phouma with Averell Harriman and Dean Rusk,
Secretary of State, in Washington, October 1967.

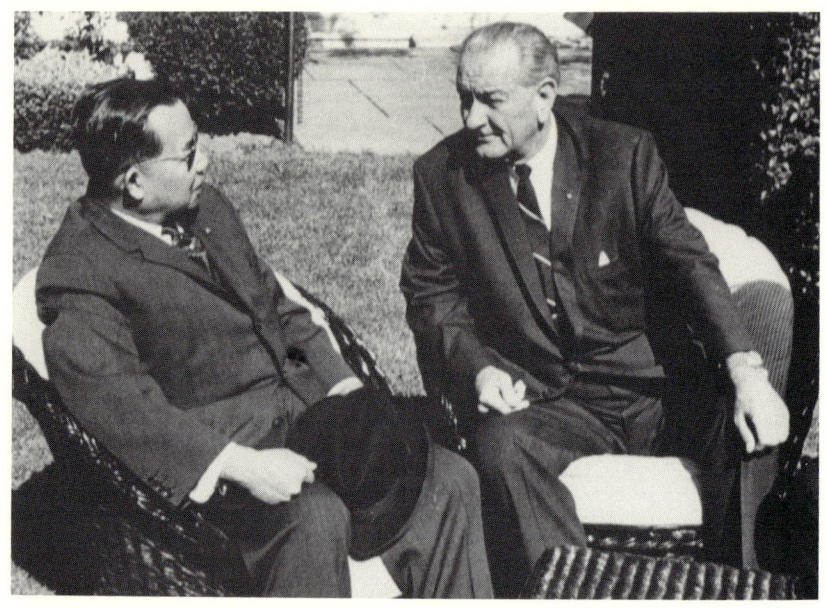

Prince Souvanna Phouma with President Johnson, The White House, 1967.

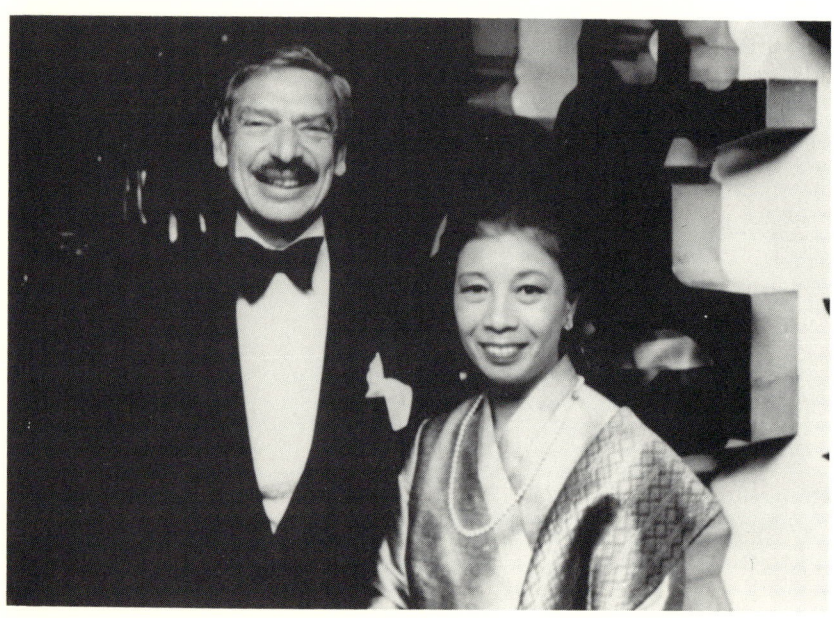

The author with his wife, Moune.

desks that are intended to support the overseas mission and, if the people there are not otherwise engaged, chatting with them about anything whatsoever.

It happened that my ten days in Washington coincided with the days of the official visit of Prince Souvanna Phouma. He was accompanied by Princess Moune, whose presence in the city was made conspicuous by a picture in the *Washington Post*.

I put through a telephone call to Blair House, where she and her father were staying and to my happy surprise succeeded in speaking with her. I told here how much I wanted to see her while she was in town—anytime she could be free. It was hopeless. The morning I called she was on her way across the street to the White House, where she would be the only woman at a small luncheon in honor of her father that was being hosted by the president with Vice President Humphrey and Governor Harriman and a few others at the table. She informed me that her schedule had no respite. Actually, she was on official duty and would make no compromise. What a serious servant of the state she was. My sole consolation was to be able to tell her that I expected to see her in Vientiane before Christmas.

At the conclusion of that White House luncheon, the president and prime minister, in traditional fashion, exchanged toasts, and their statements are duly recorded in the *State Department Bulletin*.

President Johnson in his remarks said: "The fact that the people of your brave land were able and determined to hold free elections while deeply engaged in defending themselves against armed violence, Your Highness, was a very inspiring demonstration of their resolve to control their own destiny."

The prince declared in part in his reply: "Earlier, Mr. President, you spoke of people in control of their own destiny. We certainly agree. Whatever may be said by some other powers who call us lackeys of the United States, I can proudly say that we shall never accept anything that is against our own interests. . . ."

"It is to avoid war in Laos that I have been following my policy of neutrality for almost ten years, and I am happy to see that more and more countries today share in this idea."

I was amused when I read the toasts. I thought, very good *Altesse*. You remind this country that we once opposed your government and your policy of neutrality. We should be reminded of this. We have changed. You have not.

◆ ◆ ◆

My return to Laos in December was delayed for several days by a stopover in Tokyo, where I have a good friend, a Japanese television producer. Kusi-san's wife guided me by day through the museums, but in the evening she disappeared while Kusi-san and I enjoyed bars and restaurants where Japanese businessmen obviously prefer not to have their spouses with them. And we drank much saki.

I flew to Hong Kong, checked into the Peninsula Hotel late in the evening, and woke during the night feeling extremely queasy. Too much saki, I decided. But in the morning I could not drink the tea the waiter brought into my room and had difficulty getting out of bed. How curious, I thought. I made my way down to the lobby of the hotel where a group of British doctors had offices. One of the doctors examined me, took a blood test, and informed this incredulous patient that I was to be rushed to the hospital for an appendectomy.

Days later, glum and annoyed as I tossed on my bed in a hospital run by Irish nuns and Chinese nurses, I received a cable. It came from Vientiane and read: "Your friends are deeply concerned." It was signed "Moune." I promptly got out of bed, dressed, and told the good Irish sister in charge that she would have to release me for I was leaving at once for Laos.

IV

War and Love

1967–1968

D uring that next year in Laos, I kept a journal—unwittingly as it happens.

My sister, Muriel, and I were orphaned at a relatively early age, and the closeness of our relationship was made even stronger when she married an exceptional man, Joseph Shapiro, who became my brother and my attorney, accountant, and banker. When I was overseas, we corresponded often, and from the end of 1967 through 1968 I wrote to them mostly twice a week, happy to be able to divulge very private sentiments.

Recently my sister presented me with a shoe box crammed with my letters. I had had no inkling that she had saved them. If their dominating subject is a romance, they also, it seems to me, present an intimate, however special, view of life in the capital of the little kingdom during that period.

These are selections from my letters.

◆ ◆ ◆

December 1967
Back in Laos—for me it is like a return to a favorite vacation spot.

In the nine years since I first came to this city as an apprehensive schoolteacher, both Vientiane and I have changed greatly, but underneath it all we are, I am sure, very much as we were. One change was apparent when the plane landed on Thursday afternoon and I found the ramshackle airport replaced by a quite handsome two-story affair with large glass windows. Another marked difference: those awaiting the arriving passengers are no longer allowed to walk directly out on the tarmac. And we passengers had to go through proper, albeit polite and gentle, customs.

Dave Shepperd, the new public affairs officer, and most of the USIS officers were on hand to welcome me. Dave, a Harvard man and former screenwriter, seems first rate—my kind of a person, and very different from the USIS people here when I was assigned to Savannakhet. Dave promptly told me I had surprised him. After my experience in Hong Kong, he had been expecting a hobbling convalescent.

Our drive into town filled me with nostalgia, especially as we passed those lovely *wats* and had glimpses of the saffron *bonzes* strolling across the green lawns.

I know well the house that has been assigned to me. It is the one in which John and Jean Stoddard lived. Large and with a good-sized dining room, it is unfortunately located near the morning market, and the activity of the market spills over. I recall how impossible it was in the rainy season when the road was an enormous puddle and there was no place to park the cars. I would prefer a smaller house near the river and shall see if a change in lodgings can be arranged.

A grand surprise: good, faithful Ky, who, with Mien, took such excellent care of me in Savannakhet and moved up with me to Vientiane, was waiting for me. Mien was visiting family in Saigon, but she returned yesterday with Kong, their baby, who is now a fine young fellow of seven. The house is therefore ready for me in the best sense.

Two long conversations with Dave convince me that the official American attitude toward Laos has very much improved. The threat from the Pathet Lao is, if anything, graver than it was, but we are working with the noncommunist Lao in a helpful manner. We are not being condescending toward them—nor trying to frighten them into a belligerent posture. Instead we are showing that we understand the policy of Prince Souvanna Phouma. At last!

There are, to be sure, other problems. The government is conducting its affairs with new independence. As Souvanna told President Johnson only last month, they are not lackeys of the Americans, and they fear being drawn inexorably into the affairs of South Vietnam. The French, who remain the dominant foreign friend of the kingdom, are trying to keep Laos within their own sphere of influence, and relations in Vientiane between the French and the Americans are decidedly cool.

Yesterday I checked into the embassy and met with Bob Hurwitch, the chargé while Ambassador Bill Sullivan is away. Afterwards went out to the infirmary where the American doctor looked at the scar of my operation and declared it is healing well.

I put through a phone call to Moune. She is living in her father's residence and invited me to stop by at the end of the afternoon. Amusingly enough, shortly after my conversation with her, one of my USIS colleagues, in an effort to reveal that he was well informed about me, let me know that although I may have been an occasional guest at the prime minister's house during my previous stay in this city, it was extremely unlikely that I would be invited back any time soon. "The situation," he announced, "is very different now." I refrained from telling him that I was going there that evening.

And what a warm reception I received at the residence. First Moune came downstairs, then her father, and lastly her brother Panya joined us. We sat, talked, and had drinks. We spoke of the latest developments in the relations of Laos with the United States and other countries. We discussed the growing disaster in nearby Vietnam. And we chatted about ourselves—about Paris, and Vientiane, and the prince's recent visit to Washington. What intelligent, sensitive, and gracious people the Souvanna Phoumas are. Sitting there in that long, white, high-ceilinged salon with the crystal chandeliers, I felt there was no place I would rather have been, no people I would rather have been with.

Moune is working strenuously at the Ministry of Foreign Affairs, but she looks marvelous, younger and more vigorous. Last evening I felt closer to her than I had in Paris. Yet, I must admit, as cordial as she is, she continues to possess a certain aloofness—or at least I think she does. I wonder if I shall ever be able to break that down.

And I wonder about the rumors I've heard, even when I was in Paris, that a certain Lao, young, wealthy, Western-educated, of a prominent family, with a brother who is a minister in the government, has been determinedly courting her. I know him slightly— Ph. is certainly an eligible bachelor with an agreeable personality. Furthermore, he is, I understand, on excellent terms with both the prince and the princess. No one mentioned him last evening, and I didn't think about him then, but I am wondering about him now.

Sunday Panya invited some fifty young friends, mostly Lao and French but with a scattering of Thais and Japanese and even two

Americans, out to the family country home at Nong Thevada, and Moune suggested I join the picnic party. We drove out to a large, old-fashioned, frame house, a pleasing mixture of Lao and Western architectural features. The house, though, has not been lived in in recent years and looks it. But the location on a winding river is beautiful.

The weather was pleasant—not too hot—and we wandered about. Some played volleyball, and Panya made an effort to interest a sufficient number in a bit of rugby. And the Lao food was delicious.

When Panya and his guests left, Moune and I remained for a while because the people of the house and the tiny village, servants and farmers, had asked to speak with her. Naturally, I was a keenly curious observer. Moune sat on a straw mat that had been placed on the grass for her while some twenty or so persons, men and women, few with more than a basic education, many with alert, fine-featured faces, sat on the ground in front of her. The discussion was conducted with the utmost seriousness and profound respect on both sides. They asked questions and listened intently. She provided answers and volunteered information. When the session ended, perhaps a half an hour later, Moune and her audience gracefully rose to their feet. They *waied* to her with deep reverence, she to them with charm.

I asked her about the nature of their questions as we drove back to the city. They were worried, she said, about reports that reached them of the fighting in the north of the kingdom and were especially troubled since two refugees had recently passed through the village with tales of terror. She had explained to the group what the government was doing in its efforts to establish peace. She never thought of demanding their loyalty; they were loyal. It occurred to me that when most people have the opportunity of addressing someone close to the head of state, their foremost concern might understandably be their own economic welfare, but not in the little kingdom, where material want is minimal.

I doubt that I shall ever forget seeing Moune, that ultimate example of Paris chic, a woman perfectly at ease with the world's political and society leaders, being equally at ease with and entirely considerate of her own people, including her servants.

"A paradox, a paradox, a most ingenious paradox." Am thinking about Gilbert's lyric and wondering: Can I be the good foreign service officer that I believe I am if basically I am anything but nationalistic? Although, let me say on my own behalf, I do perceive nationalistic nuances.

What brings this to mind is that I am spending far more of my free time with members of the French community than with my fellow Americans. I could say I was doing this to help Franco-American relations in this city, but that wouldn't be true. My only reason is that this is my present preference.

When Moune is busy, as she often is—and not, I hope, with Ph.—I sometimes go out with Denyse, a pleasant gal from Nice who taught at the lycée when I did and who is still teaching there. The French cultural attaché and I seemed to have formed on very short notice a warm bond of sympathy and budding friendship. And the French consul and his wife have extended to me a hearty invitation to join their French friends for late Sunday afternoon gatherings at their home where boule is played and supper served.

Now I am keenly aware that I am a representative American and that the French here as elsewhere tend to consider themselves the superior people. That old French chauvinism! When I am the only one of my country at a French get-together, I want them to realize that an American is present. At the same time, I of course want to be accepted for myself and not as a token. I will not allow an anti-American remark to pass unchallenged, but, come to think of it, no one is making anti-American remarks in my presence. And maybe I am making too much of this issue.

I suppose some of my sensitivity in this regard comes from having been brought up as a Jew in an essentially non-Jewish community where I knew both discrimination and acceptance but wished to be accepted not despite my religion but with recognition of it.

The news from up north is grim as the North Vietnamese–Pathet Lao push on. With each advance, the number of refugees grows. Poor little kingdom and its gentle people—the percentage of its population forced to flee from their villages is perhaps the highest in any country, a sad mark of distinction in this refugee-producing century.

Life in Vientiane remains more removed from the fighting in spirit than in miles. The average man here lives relatively well, while the mandarins and we diplomats spend all our evenings at cocktail and dinner parties. Not that there is indifference to the country's situation—not at all. But what to do? Sometimes I think how I eat extravagently well, live more luxuriously than comfortably, while nearby are those who are underfed and inadequately housed, and I do not share with them. It's wrong, and I know it's wrong.

Maybe I am going on in this vein because I am in danger these days of being engulfed in euphoria, and last evening was a landmark occasion. Nakhala Chounramany, of the Ministry of Foreign Affairs and a cousin of Ambassador Nouphat Chounramany of Paris, gave a dinner party at his home. You may recall my having spoken of René Weill, the French director of Radio Laos—it was he who first brought me to Prince Souvanna's residence to play bridge. René and his wife, Janine, are a witty couple, and it was fun to find them at Nakhala's. As the three of us chatted away, their dear friend Moune arrived.

Looking back at last evening, I was damned impolite—but so was Moune. From the time she arrived until she left, we tolerated René and Janine's company for a while, but otherwise we paid attention only to each other. I can understand my own behavior. Ever since I first saw Moune walk into Nouphat's house in Paris, I wished to concentrate entirely upon her. But this morning I realize that she, who I suspect does little by chance, made no objection to my monopolizing her company. This makes me cognizant of a change in our relationship—a change as I would have it.

So despite my profound sympathy, and sometimes anguish, for what is happening in this kingdom, I am a happy man, and my happiness depends upon being here.

———————

What a Christmas weekend this has been, Saturday evening, the prime minister had a small dinner party, *en famille*, to welcome me back. Prince Mangkhara and Princess Ouanna, his elder son and his lovely wife, were there. So were René and Janine Weill. With Moune, that made seven of us. Bright conversation, a delicious dinner with both Lao and French dishes, good brandy and big Havanas, and then bridge until 1:30. No event to welcome me could have pleased me more.

Last evening, Christmas Eve, I went to the home of one of my USIS colleagues but left there at ten to proceed to the French ambassador's residence. While in Paris, I had met through mutual friends Claude and Sonia Arnaud shortly before they left for Laos, where Claude is the French ambassador. He strikes me as a serious and somewhat introverted man, in sharp contrast to his exuberant and joyous South American wife. When I got there, Sonia kissed me and scolded me for not having called on her as soon as I arrived in Vientiane.

Denyse, René and Janine, the delightful Thai ambassador and his wife, and amusing Ngon Sananikone were among the thirty or so invitees, but I was the only American. Most went to the Catholic church, which is nearby, for midnight mass, leaving the Thai ambassador, the French cultural attaché, René, and myself to play a few rubbers of bridge. At one o'clock the group returned from church and with them was Moune. She, have I mentioned, was brought up a Catholic, the religion of her mother. I was a bit surprised that when Moune came in she gave me such an effusive embrace in front of all the others. More champagne, a distribution of gifts, and a *foie gras* and lobster supper. At four in the morning, in the clumsy jeep-wagon which is the only vehicle at my disposal, I drove home Denyse, and then another guest, and, last stop of course, Moune.

Understandable, isn't it, that I prefer Vientiane even to Paris.

———————

Georges Marguier, the French cultural attaché, is not only a fine fellow but he entertains the way a cultural attaché should. I was at his home for a dinner party. Most of his guests were Lao, including the minister of education, and after dinner a few Lao musicians played and we all danced that irresistible *lam vong*.

Last evening I was back at the prime minister's residence for a brief, pleasant visit with the prince, Mangkhara, and Oanna. Then

Moune and I had one of those rare evenings when we were free to be together on our own. We went to our favorite French restaurant, where for the holiday season they had a Filipino combo. There were very few patrons, and Moune and I had the dance floor to ourselves. Moune, I learned, had studied ballet, and she dances as though she had.

When we left the restaurant, we headed out to the newly developed Strip, as it is called, near the Boulevard Circulaire. Amusing—a whole line of night clubs, so unlike what Vientiane used to be. Whether this is the result of the recent hippie invasion, or whether the hippies came because the clubs were there is a chicken-or-egg question, but both are there now. The *boîte* that gets the most attention is the Third Eye—elaborate psychedelic decor, dark, dense, far-out music, where most of the customers smoke but not tobacco, and at the same time, with a sort of silly, homey atmosphere—not at all ominous. Drugs are available in this city, but the gangsters who peddle them are not. We sipped brandy, then left to get some needed fresh air.

Tomorrow is New Year's Eve, and on this occasion Prince Souvanna traditionally receives his top government officials and the senior members of the diplomatic corps at a black tie dance and reception. My rank is not high enough to be included on that list, but I nevertheless have been invited and am looking forward to spending the evening in Moune's presence.

On the last day of the year, very troubling reports reached us. A large number of Lao soldiers stationed north of Luang Prabang in an area called Nambac are apparently encircled by an even larger number of Pathet Lao and North Vietnamese soldiers. Some are remarking that the government soldiers are in a valley similar in many ways to Dienbienphu. This hardly made for a genial background for the New Year's celebration.

Since my previous stay, one major change in Vientiane has been the construction of a grand hotel, a sorely needed addition built with government funds. It is named the Lan Xang—Million Elephants—and is quite attractive and perfectly located downtown on the Mekong. There are large reception rooms and a very large terrace overlooking the river and the flame trees.

Prince Souvanna held his reception at the hotel, and despite the situation in the north, it was a gala affair. He, Moune, Mangkhara, Oanna, and Panya formed the receiving line. Hundreds of glamorously dressed invitees danced to orchestras which played on the terrace and in the ballroom and then watched a lovely performance of classical dance by those exquisite young girls of the Ecole Natasinh. We were assigned to tables, which meant that I was at a distance from Moune, who was her father's hostess. Naturally, I kept an eye on her table and managed to have a set of dances with her. I noticed that Ph. also danced with her.

The North Vietnamese chargé d'affaires was present, and I, along with almost everyone else, noticed Souvanna in conversation with him. Imagine, the enemy was there, celebrating, and being politely received. That's the way it often is in this little kingdom.

When Souvanna rose to welcome his guests, rather than offer the traditional toast, he chose to speak of the situation which threatens the country. He spoke forthrightly and, as he always does, eschewed demagoguery. But in his remarks he made it absolutely clear who was responsible for the diminishing hope for peace that the Geneva accords had promised. I was terribly moved to hear him speak of his great disappointment. He made one statement which I looked up in the next day's Lao Presse so that I could quote it to you exactly. Here it is: "Because peace is not in our hands, we must depend on the will of other nations. We are still waiting to see whether our friends who talk about peace so constantly can actually do something to bring peace to our country."

Upon hearing that, the representatives of foreign countries who were gathering in the room should damned well have felt if not a sense of guilt at least one of responsibility.

Midnight, "Auld Lang Syne," and in the crush of people seeking each other out, I shot like an arrow to you-know-who, held her in my arms, kissed her, and wished her the happiest of years.

◆ ◆ ◆

January 1968

What is happening up north in the region of Nambac has us tremendously concerned. The government has some four thousand troops there, and they are surrounded by thousands of North Vietnamese and Pathet Lao soldiers. This winter, the dry season, the Pathet Lao have been less active militarily than they usually are, that is until this recent development.

Because in this little kingdom there have been few or no major fronts in the ongoing conflict with the Pathet Lao, the sudden presence of one—and such an important and unexpected one as Nambac—is ominous.

What I am saying, however, in no way means that you are to worry about your brother here in Vientiane, unless you wish to worry that I am running myself ragged on an overactive social schedule. Furthermore, in this city we are at least subconsciously aware that should real danger thrust itself upon the scene, we are on the shores of the Mekong and just a long swim away from safety. Which suddenly leaves me to wonder if Moune is a good swimmer.

The barrier swings open, and in floats a raft of memories of graduate days at Harvard. Quite by chance, I encountered Robert Hillyer's son, Stanley, here in Vientiane. When I studied with Robert, and later would sail with him in Connecticut, he had spoken of his son, and Stanley recognized my name immediately, for his dad had spoken of me. Stanley is in town with his very attractive Italian wife, Laura, and the three of us have indulged in an orgy of reminiscing, even though this is the first time we have met.

Even more curious, the reason Stanley came to Vientiane is because he is a friend of Moune's suitor, Ph. After lunch with the three of them, I was alone with Ph. for a while in the lobby of the Lan Xang. He informed me in gentlemanly fashion that he knew I was often with Moune, did not object to that, but wanted me to understand that he was going to marry her.

I invited Stanley, Laura, and Ph. to dinner at my home. Ph. and I acknowledged that we were on good terms but that those terms are subject to change.

Our fears have been realized at Nambac. Thousands of soldiers have been forced to make a fighting retreat as the North Vietnamese–Pathet Lao military pressure expands. The Lao army has to abandon much of its munitions and equipment.

Souvanna Phouma is determined to bring a measure of calm in the wake of this northern rout and today made a statement to assure the world that the military situation in the little kingdom has not appreciably deteriorated. This courageous leader will continue his efforts to bring some sort of peace to the country.

Since I came back to Vientiane, USIS has made transportation available to me, and I do appreciate that, but the only sort of transportation USIS has to offer is a big hulk of a jeep-wagon. Fortunately, Moune is so agile and graceful that she can make even climbing up into and down from that absurdly high passenger seat an attractive maneuver, and she has never complained. But I have felt the need to change my vehicle.

Sunday morning while walking down the main street near the afternoon market, I spotted in one of the shops a bright blue Baby MG. Tiny but as pretty as can be. Open with a canvas top that can be attached in case of rain. The contrast with what I have been driving could hardly be greater, the price of the new car was considerably less than I feared it would be, and the result is I'm like a kid with a new toy.

Last evening I went to the residence to call for Moune. Her father was at home, and we had a drink together. USIS wants to do a documentary film about the prime minister for distribution throughout the country—or at least that part of the country which remains under government control. Dave had suggested that perhaps I could approach the prince on the subject. I did, and he agreed. If this is using my personal relationship for professional advantage, in an instance such as this where everyone stands to gain, I see no wrong in doing so.

Moune and I left her father to go to the French club for dinner with the Weills. When we stepped out of the house, Moune let out a squeal of pleasure at her first view of the car. At the club, René and Janine demanded to know if I had to use a lubricant to squeeze into the MG. Nevertheless, I do fit into it—very well.

On Tuesday Moune found herself without wheels, and I insisted she make use of the MG. Only later did it occur to me that that tiny car was making a big splash in this city. Not mine for much more than a week, it has already become a conspicuous object identified with its owner. By Tuesday evening, at least three persons had remarked to me that they had seen the princess darting about in my car. If I had soberly thought this over before I purchased it, I might have hesitated—probably should have hesitated—but I'm glad I didn't hesitate even if there may now be those who will say: *"L'attaché cultural américain n'est pas un homme très serieux."*

These are days with Moune and therefore blissfully happy ones. We keep finding reasons to see each other, some matter to attend to at the Ministry, or a visit to encourage a local artist, or just some something we invent. Our evenings are also spent together, except for last night when she had to attend an official dinner, leaving me to feel strangely alone although I went to both a cocktail and a dinner party.

Yesterday afternoon we went to the stadium to see the opening soccer match of the season, for which Panya switched from rugby to soccer and displayed his athletic prowess and versatility. After the match we wanted to take a spin, but Vientiane offers few scenic routes. However, we rode along the Mekong. A river that flows through tropical vegetation cannot fail to have an exotic allure.

I say that these are happy days for me, and they are. Yet I can never forget that I am enormously involved in this kingdom whose existence may, I fear, be threatened by the setback at Nambac.

Two representatives of the World Buddhist Organization are here from Sri Lanka to prepare for a conference of the organization to be held in Vientiane next year. This is expected to be an important event with delegates from all over, and assistance is needed for publicity, documentation, printing, photo coverage, film projections, and innumerable other details. The cooperation of the

American cultural services has been requested, and we are happy to provide whatever we can. Last evening I was invited to a meeting and dinner in honor of the visitors, and the ten Lao present, including two ministers, were an outstanding group.

Being with them, listening to them, observing the manner in which they conduct themselves, made me again aware of the qualities that are so evident and so admirable among the inhabitants of this little kingdom: a quiet dignity, a sense of devoutness that comes through with no superficial or hypocritical piousness, a rich sense of humor that indicates a profound understanding and acceptance of life. Compassion is there but not flaunted, and sentimentality is avoided. All of these qualities are consistent with their religion. Guided by the laws of Buddha, which are morally equivalent to our commandments, these people do not suffer the fear of damnation if they transgress. They possess instead the sadness and the comedy of knowing that no man can be without sin. And this, I presume, gives Buddhists the great sense of tolerance for which they are renowned.

Moune's boss, the director of the Ministry of Foreign Affairs, was there. An affable prince, he knows full well that I am a frequent caller at his Ministry. Last evening, with a big grin, he told me that if I wished to visit someone at the Ministry, his permission had to be obtained, and he would therefore expect me to be calling on him often.

———

We hear that those thousands of Lao soldiers who were forced to flee from Nambac are attempting to draw a new line of defense above Luang Prabang. It is vital that they succeed. As for the North Vietnamese, they continue to claim that they did not participate in the Nambac debacle, that it was the Pathet Lao alone who scored a victory. Anyone who would believe that will believe that the Soviets have granted Czechoslovakia its freedom and independence.

With many Royal Lao Army troops up north to aid their fellow soldiers, the North Vietnamese–Pathet Lao armies are making their presence more ugly in the southern part of this country. For instance, they have seized truckloads of rice meant for Vientiane and sent them off to Vietnam. Years ago when I was here, the Thai government was creating problems for Souvanna Phouma's government by keeping necessary supplies from reaching Vientiane. Now it is the North Vietnamese who try to keep produce from reaching the capital. To be a neutralist in this world requires extraordinary stamina. Neutralism has nothing to do with softness or weakness.

Saturday morning I called for Moune at the Thai residence where she and Pina Supapol, the ambassador's enchanting wife, were at the piano playing compositions for four hands. Bhanbot Supapol, the ambassador, and I were their audience. A charming concert.

Then Moune and I went to a small luncheon in honor of her father at the French residence.

In the evening there was a large formal Red Cross ball at the Lan Xang at which Prince Souvanna was the honorary patron. And so for the first part of the evening, Moune had to sit at his table, but she soon switched to the table at which I was sitting with Bhanbot Supapol and Pina Supapol and others.

Moune tells me she has to go to Bangkok to see her doctor and then, although I hope not, may have to go to France for a month or so for minor surgery.

Moune returned from her two days in Bangkok on the same plane with Ambassador Bill Sullivan. I had met him only briefly years ago while I was in Savannakhet, but when he got off the plane, where I was waiting for Moune, his greetings and remarks made it clear that he remembered me well—or else it was because Moune had been speaking to him during the flight. I was glad to see him again. He is a remarkable diplomat and a most friendly fellow.

The next day Moune and I were driving on the southern outskirts of the city, not far from the Mekong, when we saw a sign announcing a house for rent. We followed the indicated direction to a large open area where an avenue of magnificent royal bamboos led to a contemporary-style, two-bedroom California ranch house. It must be utterly unique in this kingdom. It even has a fireplace. Beyond it are fields, then rice paddies, and at a distance a small village. The house was built by an Air America pilot who used California blueprints.

Moune and I are enormously enthusiastic. This will make life in Vientiane very different. I brought Dave and the dreary USIS admin officer up to look at it. Dave thinks the house is great, the admin man thinks only of the costs involved. True, some work is required, but the American owner will build comfortable quarters in the yard for Ky and Mien and Kong, as well as a large kitchen. I will pay the expenses of having the large open brick terrace screened and roofed, converting it into an excellent representational dining room. I should be able to move in in a month.

That Moune and I were together when we accidentally discovered the house and that we reacted to it in identical fashion gives the house a very special aura.

Other news for which I am most grateful: instead of going to France, Moune will go to Bangkok for her surgery. Of course I am worried that she is going to have an operation, but if she must, I am thankful that she will be hours away rather than at a great distance.

◆ ◆ ◆

February 1968

Did I mention in a previous letter that I was expecting a visit from Philippe Krynen, son of dear friends, Jean and Jacqueline Krynen of Toulouse? Jean was assistant mayor in charge of cultural affairs and was to a large measure responsible for the enormously successful American month I organized in his city.

Philippe is a helicopter pilot with the French navy and has been serving in Tahiti. On his way back to France, knowing that I was here, he chose to stop by. He is a fine young man with a good personality and a vibrant interest in foreign cultures. One of the first days he was here, I was busy at noon and so Moune invited him home with her, where he had lunch with the prime minister. On the following day, the prince was attending special Buddhist services at the royal *wat*, and Philippe asked if he could attend. Of course he could, and he actually spent most of a day at the temple. Another day, Claude and Sonia Arnaud came to my house for lunch, and Claude realized that he had gone to school with

Philippe's father, and Sonia therefore felt she had to arrange a luncheon for Philippe at the French residence. I introduced my visitor to the pretty daughter of an American embassy officer, and he went out with her to explore more of the city.

Once while walking with him near the American embassy, we passed on ordinary two-story building with some armed soldiers casually on duty at its entrance. The military-oriented Philippe remarked that these soldiers were not in the same uniform as the others. I explained that this was because these soldiers were Pathet Lao and the building was their Vientiane headquarters and barracks.

Philippe was perplexed. "That can't be. They're the enemy. They're fighting the Royal Army."

"But that's how it is in Laos," I replied.

He remarked, "That's damned civilized."

When I took him to the airport this morning, he said he hated to leave, that this was the "most wonderful week I've ever spent," and he was determined to return. He, too, had fallen under the spell of the little kingdom.

Unusual excitement prevails in town today. A Pathet Lao lieutenant has defected and is giving the government authorities an insight into what the Pathet Lao are planning. What he is revealing is hardly surprising, but it is dire. He reports that the North Vietnamese anticipate peace negotiations in the near future—that is, they are so confident of their successful campaign against South Vietnam—and that before entering into such negotiations they want to have certain parts of Laos occupied by themselves. They are accordingly planning an attack upon the strategically important city of Saravane in southern Laos, only twenty miles to the west of the Ho Chi Minh Trail.

Prince Souvanna was sufficiently convinced by the defector's revelations to arrange to have him repeat his story to the members of the International Control Commission. Now we shall see what if anything the commission, hopelessly crippled by its Polish member and his right of veto, will do.

Most Lao, particularly in the villages, lead lives with far less sense of want than do vast populations in other, more developed countries. But Laos is a featherweight on the world's economic scale. It has no industry, it exports no more than a pittance of tin and coffee (the opium that is smuggled out is not a legitimate export), and its currency, the kip, fares miserably on the monetary market.

This came to mind today because the more than one thousand employees of USAID are on strike. In Lao fashion, it is a gentle strike—no roughness, no threats, merely an entreaty for a raise in salaries. The Americans are aware of how pitifully low their wages are and are willing to increase them, but if we do, the Lao government will be embarrassed because this would most likely precipitate a demand for a comparable increase from its own employees.

On this subject, Moune is annoyed with me, for I pay Ky and Mien more per month than she earns as a senior official in the Ministry of Foreign Affairs. Obviously, that is shockingly wrong. But few Lao are trained for household help, and the servants who come here from Saigon and the Philippines demand and receive respectable wages.

One further thought on the Lao economy: No one is apt to be so naive as to think that the United States pours millions of dollars into the kingdom each year for altruistic purposes.

Prince Souvanna has seemed a bit under the weather lately, but last evening he came to my house for a small family-type dinner party. I feel so close to the Souvanna Phouma family at this time that I may be taking too casually my visits with them. But yesterday I was reminded of just who was arriving when motorcycle police and army jeeps escorted his car to the house. Moune was with him, of course, and Panya and René and Janine Weill joined us. After dinner we played the customary rubbers of bridge. The prince was, Moune and I were delighted to note, in excellent form.

Amusing note: the British head of intelligence while commenting upon a certain local romance remarked to our chief of station (the name we give to our head of intelligence in each country) that it was a smart American ploy to have sent Stieglitz back to Laos.

Claude and Sonia Arnaud leave Laos next month to return to France, and so, in good diplomatic fashion, everyone who knows them—who has had official or social contact with them—feels obliged to entertain them with a farewell dinner, luncheon, cocktail, or whatever. It is doubtless a mark of prestige to say that you have entertained the departing French ambassador. Anyway, since Moune and I have become their dear friends, we will be included on far too many invitation lists. That should keep us overoccupied for the next many weeks.

There is a French military mission at Vang Vieng, approximately halfway between Vientiane and Luang Prabang. This coming weekend, the Arnauds are paying their last call at the mission and have invited us to join them. Never having been there, I am looking forward to the trip.

How beautiful this country is. Saturday morning, Claude, Sonia, Moune, and I in a little French military plane went up to Vang Vieng. It is a small, bustling village—a marketplace, a *wat*, and houses on stilts going off in many directions—but it is located at the foot of spectacular mountains. And what a difference nearby mountains make. I realize that is what Vientiane needs.

We stayed at the French military mission, where as was inevitable we had far too much lunch. Then we boarded a *pirogue* that spluttered up and down the river. This flowing water is an important aspect of life for the inhabitants. They fish in it, they bathe in it, and should they wish to travel up to Luang Prabang or down to Vientiane, they voyage on it. We explored two of the large caves on the banks, but not for long, for the dark, dank cavities of the earth presented too strong a contrast to the sparkling water and sunshine outside.

On Sunday morning, the officer in charge had arranged a convoy of cars to take us up into the foothills of the mountains to the villages of the Yao tribes. The villages themselves are unexceptional in appearance, but this is opium country, and the poppies, large white and purple, are abundant and magnificent. We stopped alongside a mountain stream for a picnic lunch. Mountain streams always tempt me—I want to swim in them. But I decided that on this occasion it would have been awkward to undress and plunge into the water, and so I refrained.

This is my month for traveling within the kingdom. I had to go to Savannakhet to check on the Fulbrighters, the library, and other cultural services, and spent two nights in my old house. Much less colorful than it once was, the house has been repainted and is without its wide bands of red, blue, yellow, and combinations thereof. As for the city, there seems little new development. I called on the governor—the same one who was there in my days—and had a long conversation with him. This city which was the center of the rightists' movement to overthrow the neutralist government is now concerned solely with a defense against possible Pathet Lao incursions. I visited the kind Chinese family that had been so helpful to me and saw other people with whom I had been friendly during that year, but to my disappointment, General Boun Pone was out of town.

This year two American Fulbrighters teach in Savannakhet, and I spent an evening with them and some of their Lao colleagues and school administrators. The two are fond of the Lao and are enjoying their quiet lives.

The hotel where I had stayed until my house was ready is merely seven years old but has become quite seedy. I had the impression that it has few clients these days, and what had been the Bo Pen Yang Club is a sad, unused rooftop. Of the plethora of bars whose girls entertained the American soldiers, almost none remains.

A walk along the river brought me to Phoumi Nosavan's large old house, serene and deserted. But the Mekong as it flows past brings to Savannakhet a strange sense of grandeur.

The defector who reported that the North Vietnamese were planning an attack on Saravane has been proven to be all too accurate. The North Vietnamese and Pathet Lao soldiers are definitely increasing their forces around that town.

Today the Polish member of the International Control Commission refused to allow the commission to investigate the situation. He is acting in accordance with the intransigent communist pattern. The Indian and Canadian commissioners are nevertheless hoping to go ahead with a trip to Saravane and are attempting to obtain some sort of guarantee from the Pathet Lao that they will not be fired upon.

Even if the Poles are acting under the orders of the Soviets, it is difficult not to feel a sense of fury against them, for they are absolutely scuttling the clear-cut intent of the Geneva accords.

———————

Adding to the general consternation created by the military situation in the Saravane region is the news that yesterday a Royal Air Laos passenger plane crashed between Luang Prabang and Vientiane. Moune's cousin, Prince Khamthan, was aboard. When I was a Fulbrighter, he was the president of the Mekong Society dramatic group, and I knew him well and liked him immensely. Also on the plane were the British military attaché and other diplomats and officials. In this little community, where everyone tends to know each other, an accident like this has tremendous impact.

———————

Dave Shepperd enjoys telling the following story. Two days ago at the USIS staff meeting there was a difference of opinion about a certain policy. After the meeting, Dave asked me if I could sound out some knowledgeable Lao on the subject. That afternoon I told him that I had had lunch with the prime minister and was able to give Dave the prince's opinion on the matter. No further arguments were necessary.

———————

Hanoi the other day accused Souvanna Phouma of making false allegations to justify his use of American assistance against the Pathet Lao. In response, the prince gave an interview to the correspondent from *Le Monde* and declared that the North Vietnamese had 40,000 soldiers in Laos. He went on to say that he had enlisted American aid only when the situation within his country was sharply deteriorating.

We have every reason to believe that his stated figures are no exaggeration and wonder how long the little kingdom can continue under these conditions.

I have moved into my new home. It is a most attractive inside-outside house in a delightful rural setting. I've slept in it for two nights and find it much quieter and cooler than in the city. Best of all, Moune says she would love to live in it. Obviously, there is nothing I want more than to have her do just that.

The long anticipated North Vietnamese–Pathet Lao attack on Saravane took place this week, and it is with great relief that we hear the government forces have beaten it off. The enemy had seized a small outpost near the city, but even that has been retaken within two days. Attopeu, another strategic southern town, was also under seige, but there, too, the enemy was repelled.

For the moment, the little kingdom is alive and kicking. Hallelujah!

◆ ◆ ◆

March 1968

General Westmoreland's assessment of the Vietnam war as it appears in *The New York Times* dismays me. He is about to demand an increase in the number of American soldiers—a dreadful idea—and he states that the Vietcong morale is rapidly deteriorating, which I strongly doubt. The more we know about what is happening in Vietnam, the less confidence I have in the general.

All of this makes me grateful that I am not participating in the murky morass of Vietnam, where South Vietnamese leadership is less than inadequate and where we are conducting an undeclared war—a dangerous and highly questionable policy. Here in Laos the issues are clear-cut. This is a peaceful country whose superb leaders are elected, and although it is struggling for its existence against the North Vietnamese, it has refused the proposal to have American soldiers fight on its soil. Instead, it tries to rely on the promises made to it by the nations at Geneva.

If as a consequence of Vietnam the great powers neglect the little kingdom, it may be tragedy on a small scale, but it will be tragedy nevertheless.

Moune and I spent the weekend at home—as lovely a weekend as I have ever known. All of my Paris household effects have been unpacked in the new house. We therefore listened to records and hung pictures. Moune is just as ardent and exigent a picture hanger as you and I are. The long wall that extends from the living room through the small sitting room sports thirteen paintings, lithos, and etchings, including two Picassos, two Chagalls, a Miró, a Vertes, a Renoir, two Cézannes, and that handsome Anita de Caro. On the wall jutting out from the fireplace, the two large Braque prints are elegant, and Muriel's handsome painting of the seated figure hangs by itself between the front door and the window. My collection of Baroque records never sounded better.

Moune has become so enamored of the house she is claiming it's the house, not me, she's primarily interested in.

Tonight the Rotary Club's international film festival begins. Prince Souvanna was to have been the honorary patron, but since he is out of town, Moune has been asked to replace him. For the festival, I was able to obtain a print of *Lolita* as the American entry.

The little blue MG seems to have acquired a fame of its own. We were at the British residence for a dinner party for twenty-four persons presided over by Beryl Smedley, the ambassador's sweet and thoughtful wife. Suddenly the season's first rainstorm struck, and it was fierce. Beryl jumped up from the table, hurriedly crossed to me, and demanded the keys for the car in order to have her chauffeur drive it into the garage and protect it from the downpour.

After dinner we were all invited to see the British entry at the film festival, and since it was still raining, Moune and I were given a ride by the new Indian ambassador and his wife. The film was Fonteyn and Nureyev in the ballet version of *Romeo and Juliet*. I thought it was a bore, full of posturing and little dancing.

Lolita sold out the house and played to an enthusiastic audience. Imagine, Nabokov a smash hit in Vientiane!

At it again. The North Vietnamese and Pathet Lao soldiers are once more attacking Attopeu, this time with mortars. More than a dozen civilians have been injured, some of them gravely.

However, the Lao Air Force has been able to counterattack and apparently has inflicted casualties among the enemy.

I know killing in any form is loathsome—a sentiment I share with the Buddhists—but this country is fighting for its survival, and I'm glad to know the enemy is paying a toll for its belligerence.

You have probably read that Anthony Eden has come forth with a proposal for the neutralization of much of Laos, a neutralization to be guaranteed by the Geneva treaty signatory nations. The problem is that the treaty itself was supposed to have guaranteed neutrality for the kingdom, and this has been uninterruptedly violated by the communist forces. But if the Earl of Avon can come up with some new way of making it work, we have little to lose and much to gain.

Sonia Arnaud invited herself up to inspect the new house. She is a former decorator and difficult to please, but she was more than generous in her comments. When she learned that we were having problems such as getting nails into the walls, she, without asking us, sent the French embassy's supervisor and assistants to the house to take care of such details. Then yesterday the French embassy's gardener arrived to do some landscaping.

No wonder even I get confused as to which embassy I belong.

I was leaving the bar of the Lan Xang early Friday evening when I saw at the hotel's registration desk none other than the doyenne of American letters, Mary McCarthy. I'm sure I told you that while in Paris I had met Mary on several occasions, knew professionally her husband, Jim West, and had been to their apartment. I have great admiration for the woman—used to urge the girls at Hunter to read her superb *Memories of a Catholic Childhood*—and was enormously pleased to find her in Vientiane.

Mary had come here on her way to Hanoi. The International Control Commission operates a biweekly flight between the two cities, but the schedule becomes erratic in practice, and when Mary arrived she learned that she would have to wait until today, Tuesday, for her connecting flight. She is going to Hanoi as the guest of the North Vietnamese government, news that saddened me, but not enough to keep me from extending hospitality. And then this seemed an opportunity to make Mary as knowledgeable as possible about the situation in the little kingdom.

I invited Mary to have lunch with Moune and me on Saturday. She readily accepted, and since she is traveling with a mathematics professor from Berkeley, I included him in the invitation.

They arrived at the house, and Moune and I learned that until this trip Mary had never met her traveling companion, about whom she seemed ill at ease. She had reason to be. Conversation at the table made me wish I had never met him. Of German Jewish refugee background, he has become hysterically involved in protests because he is convinced that we, the United States, are destroying and killing the innocent North Vietnamese. We are guilty of waging an undeclared war against them, and I wish we weren't, but damn it, they are anything but innocent, and anyone who insists they are merely victims insists out of ignorance. In addition to his unacceptable viewpoint, I found him to have an unpleasant personality.

Despite this, Moune and I enjoyed having Mary with us. She was interested in what we had to say about Laos and asked pertinent questions. The professor was cynical about the proclaimed neutrality of the kingdom. When I was alone with Mary for a few moments, she commented about Moune in glowing terms. She also suggested that our mutual friends in Paris would be happy to hear about my relationship with Moune. I told her it was important not to reveal anything for the present.

That evening, Saturday, Sonia was having a huge charity affair. She converted the lawns of her residence into lavish fairgrounds, and some eight hundred persons paid their tribute to charity and to Sonia. I suggested that Mary and the professor might wish to attend, and they did. But he either had had too much to drink or was under too much stress. I greeted them near the gate and walked with them up the path to where Ambassador Sullivan was speaking to some others. I presented Mary to Bill and then introduced the professor, who spluttered out some obscene remarks about American policy and then, with all of us watching, swung at Bill. Our ambassador is a spry man who could more than hold his own in a physical combat with this ungainly academic, but several of us jumped into the fray to separate them. Mary was, as you can imagine, terribly upset. I asked her to wait with Moune, apologized to Bill, and escorted the would-be pugilist out to the gate and into a pedicab, instructing the driver to deposit him back at the hotel.

All of Mary's doubts were now confirmed. She was going to Hanoi, an idea which made her somewhat uneasy, with an unstable man. Moune and I tried to keep her occupied and introduced her to many people at the fair, including Sonia. But we understood that Mary did not wish to remain long after her all too spectacular entrance.

We had Mary back to the house for lunch yesterday, Monday. By herself. This gave us the opportunity to speak at greater length about the situation of this kingdom. We were pleased and grateful when she volunteered to discuss Laos with the Hanoi minister of foreign affairs, whom she was expecting to meet. And in the afternoon, Moune arranged for Mary to spend half an hour with Prince Souvanna.

For her last evening in town, Mary invited Moune and me to

have dinner with her at the hotel. Moune had an official engagement, but I had a most pleasant dinner with Mary. We talked literature, not politics, and she is so supremely expert on literature and culture and sociology that I wish she would remain within her fields of great expertise and not stray off as an expert in international politics. I say this because in spite of her brilliance and the sympathy toward Laos she is now expressing, she, too, I fear, has been taken in by the North Vietnamese protestations of innocence. To condemn what we are doing is a far cry from confusing aggressors and victims.

As we were finishing dinner, Arnaud de Borchgraves of *Newsweek* and Keyes Beech of the *Chicago Daily News* spotted Mary and suggested we go to the Strip for a drink or two. Mary agreed, and the four of us set off. We stopped at the Third Eye and then at another, quieter bar in order to hear ourselves argue. And argue they did. Arnaud is very much of a political rightist and a hawk on the Vietnam issue. Mary, I suppose, would have to be classified as a fluttering dove. Keyes sides with Arnaud but was a gentleman about it. Arnaud got real tough—even abrasive—and for the second time during her brief visit to this city I thought Mary was about to become involved in fisticuffs, this time aimed at her.

It was disturbing. Here are two exceptionally intelligent and well-informed Americans with a vehement, basic difference about our international policy. What is more, I don't agree with either of them. Sending vast numbers of our soldiers to Vietnam has been a grievous mistake—and I have felt this since the inception of Johnson's policy. But never for an instant could I fail to recognize that the devastation of Indochina has been caused by the ruthless North Vietnamese, who are absolutely responsible for the horrendous mess.

The plane for Hanoi left today, and Mary will be coming back through Vientiane. Moune and I hope to see her then and hear what she had to say to the foreign minster.

But here is a bit of news that is of greatest importance to me. Late Sunday evening I called for Moune at the prime minister's house and found myself alone with him. He had a bottle of champagne opened, and as we drank I told him what he already knew—that I was madly in love with his daughter and wished to marry her. He was beautiful and kind about it—reminded me that he had known me for many years and said simply that if Moune and I were happy together he would extend his blessings to our union.

My extreme happiness that day was, however, tempered by my conversation with Moune that afternoon. She has been impatiently expecting her divorce decree from Paris. She had not received it and the letter which reached her on Saturday suggested possible complications in the divorce court. She is deeply disturbed by this. In addition, she has set an early April date for the surgery at the Bangkok Nursing Home.

Am so glad I brought with me the recording of *Once Upon a Mattress*. In it is my favorite song. Its lyrics are:

> For a princess is a delicate thing,
> Delicate and rare as a dragon-fly's wing.
> You can tell a lady by her elegant air,
> But a genuine princess is exceedingly rare.

Minister of Finance Sisouk na Champassak and his French wife Christiane gave a farewell dinner party for Claude and Sonia. It was relatively intimate and gave me a chance to have a rather long after-dinner discussion with Sisouk. His past association with Phoumi Nosavan had long made me somewhat suspicious of him, but I am now convinced that he has come very much into his own and is the true heir—that is, politically—to Prince Souvanna. Sisouk was always a devoted Lao patriot, but slowly he has come to the realization that neutrality presents the only possible way for the kingdom's survival. One cannot doubt that he will fight and sacrifice if necessary to protect the continued existence of his country. He is a dynamic national leader, and it is reassuring to think that Souvanna has a Sisouk to count on.

Flora Lewis, of *Newsweek* and the *Washington Post*, was here two weeks ago and interviewed Moune. I've always respected Flora's keenly analytical style and never more so than today as I read her column in the *Post*, which begins: "Princess Moune lives up to her name, a young woman of serene beauty. But she is more than decorative. She is chief assistant to her father, Prince Souvanna Phouma, Prime Minister of Laos, and her mind is as cool and as clear as her voice." Flora then goes on to discuss the situation in this country. Such columns will, I hope, help people understand what is happening in Laos.

Happy to know that Johnson is withdrawing himself as a candidate in the next election. This could help us find a way to proceed in our ghastly involvement in Vietnam. I would also hope that Hubert Humphrey does not run for the presidency. His own statements on the war should certainly defeat him at the polls. They make me, who once admired him, not want to vote for him.

◆ ◆ ◆

April 1968

This past weekend, with Moune's mother still in Paris, her father was at home by himself. Moune and I therefore spent a large part of the weekend with him at his residence. Just the three of us had dinner together Saturday evening and lunch on Sunday. I made some sort of would-be witty comment about having become a boarder, but the prince replied warmly that he is happy to have me take my meals with him and wants me to do so regularly. I felt, and should have felt, enormously complimented.

In this city with its intensive social life, any host or hostess would be flattered to receive the prince. He enjoys social events and adds luster to them. But he accepts few invitations. He has many friends, but he cannot afford to have cronies in the ordinary sense. Like a man who is engaged in writing a serious work of literature, he must spend long hours in solitary reflection. He is aware that every action he takes, every decision he makes, will have beneficial or deleterious consequences for Laos.

Nevertheless, I believe he is at ease with his terrible responsibility and suspect there is little about which he feels guilty. And why should it be otherwise? He is a devout Buddhist and acts in accordance with high ethical principles. He rarely displays any trace of arrogance. He has mastered both Eastern and Western political wisdom—his stubborn insistence upon the democratic process of elections is an example of the latter.

Not that I mean to imply that he is saintly. Not at all. He has a temper, and I have seen him when he is furious with his enemies and once in a while annoyed with his children. However, these outbursts are infrequent. Almost all of the time he is clothed in a wholly natural dignity.

Moune is, I believe, the person closest to him. He loves her dearly, and she him. But she has been brought up to respect her parents, and she does. Whether working with him, as she often does, or serving as his hostess at a social function, she is the dutiful daughter.

That Prince Souvanna accepts me as a close family member touches me deeply. There is, to be sure, a lack of the casual American-style informality. For instance, when we are at the table, he insists that I, as a guest in his house, am served before he is. I have protested to no avail. Yesterday, at lunch, I said: "*Altesse,* after Moune and I are married, I shall insist that you are served first." He laughed.

Mary McCarthy has returned from Hanoi. Moune and I were at the airport to greet her, and we had drinks with her at the hotel. She told us that she had spoken to several North Vietnamese officials about Laos. Let us hope they listened to her.

On that same day, this week's *Time* arrived in town, and its People column carries an item about Mary's math professor throwing flabby punches at Bill Sullivan.

Wonderfully encouraging news from Paris. Moune's divorce should be final by June or July. We hate waiting—never would have believed I'd be so impatient to be married. After the wedding, we'll take a short trip back to the States in order to have you meet. How lucky you are to be acquiring such a marvelous sister-in-law.

I had to speak to Bill Sullivan about our plans for this reason: I as a foreign service officer cannot marry a foreigner without first getting permission from Washington. Actually, I have had to submit my resignation, which will be accepted if my wife-to-be fails to meet official approval. But who would say no to Moune? Bill, who has known her well since their days in Geneva, congratulated me enthusiastically and assured me he would write a letter demanding immediate approval. I have been fortunate that Bill has been ambassador during this period. Many another might well have resented my close association with the prime minister and his family.

———————

The Southeast Asia Treaty Organization has exciting prospects— if it doesn't get bogged down in petty disputes. That former colonies in this part of the world are enjoying their independence in wholly responsible fashion and meeting on equal terms with old colonial powers is already a fine accomplishment. Their ministers are in conference at present in New Zealand, and Secretary Rusk in an address to them has pronounced his keen disappointment with the violations of the accords on Laos established at the Geneva conference. Apparently no disagreement among the ministers exists on this issue.

I wish the little kingdom were in position to join SEATO.

———————

I've just returned from Bangkok, where I was with Moune when she checked into the hospital. The doctor is pleased with the way the surgery went, but these have been uncomfortable days for her. Moune is not, however, complaining.

Her room at the Bangkok Nursing Home has a balcony that overlooks a wooded stream. It seems very remote from the nearby honking city. The day after the operation, her visitors started to queue up—they included ambassadors and generals. The room soon became overcrowded with flowers, mostly huge baskets of variously colored and sized orchids that the Thais—and I—like so much. But the orchids are easier to admire when they are not in such profusion.

Before I left, Janine Weill arrived to remain with Moune for a few weeks. When Moune has sufficiently recovered, she and Janine will go to a guest house on the grounds of the king of Thailand's mountain residence above Chiang Mai and remain there another week or more.

One item I accomplished while in Bangkok—I went to see Alex, whose dazzling jewelry shop close to the Oriental Hotel I have frequented ever since my first visit to that city. I selected from among the rings he has designed a pale blue sapphire set on a Baroque spay of small diamonds. Alex is going to the nursing home to make sure of the finger size, and Janine will bring the ring to Vientiane with her.

As a Fulbrighter, I sometimes taught an English class for the *bonzes* at the Lao American Association. I'm fond of the old LAA building, an old colonial affair with a wooden balcony that winds its way along two sides of what had been a marketplace and is now a large, sometimes functioning fountain. All very picturesque. Our building has never made me envious of the tall, modern, uninteresting French cultural center on the other side of the fountain.

But as cultural attaché, I am involved in the planning and building of a big new LAA structure just beyond the French center. We are spending much money on this project, and as a result there will be many more classrooms and a good-sized auditorium. This will be advantageous, but I suspect I'll feel some nostalgia for the seedy old building we're abandoning.

Everyone wants to be in Luang Prabang for the Pi Mai, the Lao New Year's festival. Since I was able to go in my official capacity, I went even though I was unhappy to be without Moune. But what a memorable few days I have just spent.

Luang Prabang—more like a town than a city—must surely be one of the loveliest spots on earth. It is situated on a narrow, lush strip of ground between two rivers in a tropical, mountainous countryside. Perched on top of a tall hill in the middle of the town is a tiny, ancient temple, from which a path descends to the king's riverside palace, an unpretentious, spacious structure.

I checked into the USIS residence, where a bed had been reserved for me. There is only one hotel, the Bungalow, and its rooms are doled out to the diplomatic missions for this holiday. Then, having a little spare time, I walked along the river to see again my favorite temple in all this world, Wat Xieng Thong. It is a small, ancient wooden *wat* framed by trees laden with white, pink, and red flowers. Its roof is an intricate series of descending eaves, each ending in a delicate upturned curve. The columns holding up the roof are painted in rhythmic abstractions, and between them in the front facade are curved arches sculpted in twirls. The walls themselves are covered by dark red and faded gold carvings depicting flowers, angels, animals, and prayer. Within the dimly lit interior, a Buddha sits serenely. Nothing made by man has ever captivated me quite the way this small *wat* does.

For the first day of the celebration, a festive air prevailed. Groups of informal musicians, playing the *khen*, the flute, and the *tambour*, paraded about. On the beach, youngsters built in the sand large replicas of *stupas*, including Tat Luang, and decorated them with brightly colored ribbons. I saw people and children with cages stop to open the cage and allow the small birds captured within fly to freedom.

The most popular ceremony of the day is the water rite, and everyone seems to indulge in it. Boys and girls, men and women, take every available container, from silver bowls to crude buckets, fill them with water from the Mekong, then chase after each other and splash all in their range. Each splash is accompanied by the laughter of those who douse and those who get soaked.

As we were walking along the beach in wet clothes, a boat was hauled up, and a tall, powerful man, probably in his late thirties, debarked. He wore a white jacket and trousers, but his face was marked with lines of black paint. I recognized the crown prince. He strode up the beach, laughing gaily. Soon His Royal Highness was thoroughly drenched and laughed heartily. All who spotted him wished to have the good fortune that would come from throwing water on him.

The next morning, the atmosphere was different. This was the day of religious processions. From each *wat*, the head monk was borne on an elaborately decorated gilt palanquin. Each of these was followed by lines of *bonzes*, and after them, girls in their Lao costumes, carrying parasols to shield them from the sun. Musicians were part of each column, all conveying an aura of peace and joy.

The principal procession started from the palace. First came the royal guards in pointed scarlet helmets, gold-trimmed scarlet jackets, and dark silk dhotis that resembled eighteenth-century court breeches. The royal musicians played as the king and queen stepped out, with attendants balancing tall, tall parasols over the royal heads. Then on a palanquin came the golden Phra Bang Buddha, the statue of Buddha that is the protector of the city. The guards in red, Their Majesties and court officials in bright white, the *bonzes* in saffron—all proceeded in formation to the royal *wat*.

Folk dances were performed in the temple courtyard. Dancers wearing huge and vivid lion and dragon masks pranced about and engaged in lavishly stylistic battles. The tempo of the music accelerated, and crowds of children watched with awe, delight, or fear.

The golden Buddha was placed atop a myriad of flowers. A dragon-shaped painted conduit extended down from a high platform to a point directly over the Buddha. First the king, then the queen, climbed ladders to the platform. Each in turn poured water from great silver bowls into the conduit, and the water flowed down upon the Buddha in a ritual bath.

Tradition demands that in the afternoon one pay a pilgrimage to the grotto of Buddhas on the Mekong. The hour's travel north is in *pirogues* with outboard motors. As we made our way up the river, the green mountains, the small islands, the passing boats, and the few villages were entrancing.

The grotto is on the side of a mountain. Steep flights of white-washed stone steps climb to its entrance. In the interior, one can discern incredibly long lines of fine old Buddhas. I became absorbed in studying the differences among them, the ways in which their arms, hands, legs, feet, and torsos were positioned and the expressions of their faces.

That evening, to conclude the celebration, guests were invited to the king's palace. A platform for the royal family was at the far end, adjacent to the palace. In the middle of the courtyard was another platform for musicians and dancers. On either side were sections of seats delineated for the various groups of invitees—the government ministers and officials, the diplomats, the journalists, and the public at large.

As I was entering the grounds, Mangkhara saw me and asked me to sit with the family. I laughed and told him not yet, not this year. I sat with the diplomatic corps and watched my future in-laws assemble on the royal platform.

The lights in the courtyard were dimmed, and we all turned to face the ancient temple on top of the nearby hill. Flickering lamps softly illuminated the *wat*. As the musicians played, a line of gentle, bouncing lights started to descend the hill. This line zig-zagged, as though on a path, but grew in length, always extending from the temple. Gradually we could make out what it was we were watching: a procession of lanterns, hundreds of lanterns coming down the hill single file. When they started across the palace grounds, we could see that each was being held aloft by a Lao maiden with an angelic smile.

I doubt that any wine, any hallucinatory drug, could create a comparably magnificent sensation.

The joys of the Pi Mai are being undermined by the New Year's address Prince Souphanouvong delivered in his region in the northern part of the kingdom. He gloats over the Pathet Lao advances and proclaims that newer and bigger attacks against the government forces are underway. His troops are again hitting Attopeu and Saravane. But what he refuses to admit is that his troops could not exist at all without the full backing of the North Vietnamese army.

I've probably mentioned to you that I had met Souphanouvong several times in the old days in Vientiane. On one occasion I had dinner and played bridge with him. He presents himself as a gentleman with some of the airs of his elder half-brother—at least, he assumes those airs. If one did not know him well, one would be apt to find him quite likable. But the man is a traitor to his king and kingdom.

Imagine, he is going to be my uncle. Amusing—or perhaps not so amusing—thought: I shall be the only member of the American Foreign Service to have a prominent communist leader as an uncle.

Prince Souvanna has returned from Luang Prabang. I went past his house and we had a few whiskeys. He had caught a bad cold up north and explained that it had not helped to have had to sit on the temple floor for hours during religious ceremonies.

The absent Moune arranged a surprise birthday party for me. I was invited out for cocktails, and when I returned to my house, fifteen friends were waiting for me. The tables were set for dinner, but when René, who, at Moune's request had made the arrangements, asked Ky to serve the dinner, Ky and Mien looked at him horrified. They had not prepared the food; they had understood that it was being brought to the house. There was much laughter. Capable Josie Cader, the French consul's wife, dashed off to her house and returned within twenty minutes with the makings of a remarkably good French dinner, a conserved cassoulet that had been waiting for just such an occasion.

This is Vientiane. A situation which could have created much embarrassment back home is treated here as a good joke.

Princess Souvanna Phouma has returned from France, as grand and as exuberant as ever. Any qualms I might have had vis-à-vis her reaction to her daughter's forthcoming marriage were quickly dispelled as she warmly embraced me.

She arrived the day before the annual celebration of the Queen of England's birthday at the British embassy. This year the huge party, I was amused to note, seemed as though it had been given to welcome Princess Souvanna back to Vientiane. She was indisputably the center of attraction.

By great good fortune, the American air attaché is going to Chiang Mai tomorrow on a mission, and I will be able to fly there with him. This means I shall celebrate Moune's birthday with her, and, best of all, she is sufficiently recovered to return to Vientiane with us three days from now.

———————

Chiang Mai to me is the Thai version of Luang Prabang. Larger than LP, but not too large, it, too, is on a river with a mountain backdrop, and it contains the loveliest temples of Thailand. Chiang Mai has, I believe, far more of a Buddhist spirit than does Bangkok.

We could hardly have had a happier birthday. I presented Moune with the ring. She loves it—I love her—and we are formally engaged.

And her radiant smile informs me how glad she is to be back in Vientiane and to spend time in our house.

———————

The presence in this city of Moune's mother does somewhat dampen our style. The princess demands discretion, and therefore Moune cannot spend as much time at the ranch house as she should like.

The princess asked me to come to see her on Friday afternoon. We had tea at the residence, and then her chauffeur drove us to the outskirts of the city to a handsome and well-tended *wat*. Waiting for us was the venerable *bonze*, the royal soothsayer. It seemed not at all incongruous that the princess, a Catholic, should take me, a Jew, to heed the advice of a Buddhist sage.

The monk was younger than I had expected him to be—or perhaps he only looked young, as is often the case in this part of the world. But there was no question that he was intelligent and gentle, also outgoing. A sense of goodwill permeated. The princess and I sat with him for some time and spoke about different matters. I answered several questions about my background. Then he made his predictions in a simple, direct manner. He foresaw some immediate difficulties, but none major, and said they would be overcome. He foretold a long and happy future for Moune and myself and instructed us to follow a Lao custom, the one that I saw being observed in Luang Prabang, but in a very precise way: on the morning of our wedding day, we are to purchase small birds and fish, numbering twice our combined ages, and release the birds in the air and the fish in the river. Then we are to plant two young banana trees in close proximity to each other.

As we drove back to the city, the princess wondered if the difficulties the *bonze* had referred to might concern Moune's divorce from the Count de G. He is causing new problems in Paris.

◆ ◆ ◆

May, June, July 1968
Susan Sontag came to the house last evening. She and the journalist Andrew Kopkind and a professor from Cornell have been invited to North Vietnam as guests of the government and are in Vientiane to take the ICC plane to Hanoi. But the plane, as it often is, is delayed, and consequently they are spending several days at the Hotel Lan Xang. Mary McCarthy had suggested Susan call me.

I invited the three travelers to our home for dinner. I had hoped that Moune could make such people aware of the situation in the little kingdom, the extent of the North Vietnamese incursion. They then might, as Mary did, speak about Laos in Hanoi. In this instance, we wasted our efforts.

I had never met Miss Sontag before, but I have read and enjoyed some of her writings and looked forward to this occasion. She, however, walked into the house with a decidedly condescending attitude, and the ambience did not improve when we launched into political discussions. You know that I freely admit that we Americans have made and are making enormous mistakes in our international policies, particularly in Vietnam. But I could never engage in what sounded like an outright condemnation of America itself.

What is most troubling is that Sontag, apparently through her sorrow and anger with her own country's engagement in an undeclared war, is bestowing her sympathy upon the North Vietnamese. How can anyone who knows anything about Southeast Asian history commit such a blunder? The North Vietnamese began the conflict, they continue the conflict, and they will exploit the Soviets, the Chinese Communists, or the American intellectuals if it will help them in their century-old desire to conquer Southeast Asia.

One moment that will linger occurred when Susan looked through our collection of records, which are preponderantly of Baroque music. She turned to Kopkind and asked if he, too, remembered those days when this period music was "our" music. She clearly implied that she was sorry for those of us who did not realize that Baroque music was "out." Moune and I had a hearty laugh about that later—much later, for a tremendous rainstorm left our guests stranded at the ranch house until one o'clock this morning. I suspect they were as eager to leave as we were to bid them farewell.

(*Note*: Susan Sontag's book, *Trip To Hanoi*, was published in 1969. In it, after some eighty pages of praise for North Vietnam and criticism of the United States, she writes of her return to Vientiane and describes in some detail the taxi ride from the airport to the hotel. She observed "servile, aggressive pedicab drivers," although the Lao pedicab drivers are known to be unusually pleasant and gentle. She saw many "Cadillacs driven by American businessmen and Laotian government officials," but there were at most two Cadillacs in the city, and no more than a half-dozen American businessmen. She "passed the movie theaters showing skin flicks for the GIs"—which is the most remarkable of all because the Lao culture would never permit such films to be shown, and the American soldiers, the GIs of whom she writes, had left Vientiane fully five years before Sontag arrived. Her taxi, she claimed, then drove past the American embassy—and by the inclusion of the embassy on this list we are led to assume that the sight of it revolted her in the same way as did that of the pedicab drivers, Cadillacs and GIs. However, our embassy in Vientiane is on a side street, and it is entirely unlikely that a taxi en route from the airport to the hotel would have passed it.

We read this passage incredulously. We wondered why this intelligent, clever woman should harbor a dislike—or hatred—for gentle, little Laos so intense that she wrote about it not at all the way it was—or the way any objective person would have described it—but as she had imagined or wanted it to be. Was she unable to accept Laos being the victim of the beloved North Vietnamese? Did she want the little kingdom to welcome the North Vietnamese in as conquerors? Now that the North

Vietnamese have made Laos into one of their colonies, does that satisfy Miss Sontag's sense of justice and freedom?)

The rainy season is upon us with a vengeance—positively muddy. In the past, its arrival has been accompanied by a sharp diminution of communist attacks against the government, but this year those in the know predict that the fighting will go on almost unabated. The Pathet Lao–North Vietnamese forces are stronger and better organized than in the past. The government, however, carries on courageously.

Here's another aspect of my bride-to-be. Last evening we had a small dinner party at which the American air attaché and his good wife, Ann, were present. From the time I came back to Laos, Ann noticed the gleam in my eye whenever I glanced in Moune's direction and then did what she could to encourage the romance. She even involved—or perhaps commanded—Paul, her husband, to assist. We therefore feel something akin to indebtedness toward them.

By one o'clock this morning, Paul, an old military type close to retirement, had had a fair share of whiskey and chose, in the midst of a discussion, to proclaim his marked preference for the Phoumi Nosavan regime as opposed to the present government. As you might imagine, his comment caught the attention of everyone in the room, and a certain silence fell. But Moune, hardly missing a beat, told him without raising her voice that if he ever again uttered such sentiments, our friendship was at an end. To the extent of which he was capable, Paul tried to backtrack, and the party continued.

Moune did not permit such remarks to go unchallenged, which is natural. But she told off a friend in unmistakable terms without giving way to an emotional outpouring. She is always a lady.

What a truly international family the Souvanna Phoumas are. They are entirely at home with all that the East and the West offer. I thought of it again at Sunday lunch when the prince and princess, Mangkhara, Panya, Moune, and I were at the table. Here was the menu: smoked salmon from Scotland, *laap*, a spicy but delicious Lao version of steak tartare, Italian veal and pasta, Roquefort cheese, and local fruit, all accompanied by good French wines.

The National Assembly of Laos voted today and reelected Phoui Sananikone as its president. In this election only Assembly members participate, and Phoui defeated Prince Boun Oum's brother. The prince from Champassak attracted a good many votes on the basis of the old rightist argument that this government is not acting firmly enough against the communists. Phoui had at one time been very much to the far right in internal politics, but in recent years has given his support to Souvanna. Today's voting therefore involved an ideological dispute which ended with a victory for the moderates.

I know that family counts for too much in Laos. Phoui is a mandarin, his opponent a member of southern royalty. And not only in politics but elsewhere, one sees the heritage factor. In the military one of the leading generals is a Sananikone, another is an Abhay. One could, I suppose, argue that this kingdom is an oligarchy.

However, at national elections, the people do vote for these men as their leaders. The government is not imposed; it is popularly chosen. The government does not repress the people. It functions for their benefit. The members of the great families of the little kingdom do seem in many instances to be the best trained to assume a ruling role.

Futhermore, these men who rule are not apt to abuse their positions, or to be primarily interested in serving for monetary. This is unlike such outsiders who attained power as Phoumi Nosavan and his sidekick, Siho. But, of course, there are countless exceptions.

A thought for today is that if this is an oligarchy, maybe this is a concept worth emulation in some parts of our world.

Yesterday Moune received a cable from her lawyer in Paris which informed her that the divorce proceedings are off track. The Count of G., having learned of Moune's wish to remarry, is creating obstacles, and French law favors the husband. Moune had expected the divorce to be final by now, and this news means a possibly long delay in our plans.

We had been invited to a dinner party, but when I went to call for Moune she was not physically well enough to go out. She was suffering from a severe migraine, the result, unquestionably, of that cable. We spent a quiet and somewhat depressed evening at home.

Do you know the music of Charles Lloyd? I did not, but now that I do, I am not apt to forget it. The Charles Lloyd Quartet was sent here as a State Department cultural offering. They arrived on Tuesday, and turned out to be pure flower people, sweet, loving hippies. They play beautifully. I who am often indifferent to jazz can listen to them in complete fascination. Lloyd himself has had a classical music education, and it shows. He plays the flute and composes most of their music. It is far-out, psychedelic stuff, with much dissonance and a sense of spontaneity. It is not easy music, and his long variations on themes send some members of the audience out during each performance. I suspect that is probably true wherever he plays.

What was evident is that he struck a most responsive chord among the young Lao. The students listened to the quartet with rapt attention, and greeted them with tremendous applause. I feel certain that there is far more kinship between Lloyd's music and Lao music than between most American music and the native music of this kingdom.

I overscheduled the group, but I could not resist. On Tuesday, I hardly gave them a chance to wash up before rushing them out to the would-be university just outside the city, where they played before some fifteen hundred wildly demonstrating young Lao. The USIS camera crew was filming, and little kids were climbing all over the stage, but Lloyd and his group played on oblivious to the surrounding confusion.

The next evening we took over the auditorium of the National School of Dance, and the group performed before a cheering audience.

The following day we flew up to Luang Prabang. Moune was unable to join us—she was working on some urgent official matters. In LP, the concert at the large theater with another capacity audience was under the patronage of the crown prince, who had his special seat placed on a rug in the front row. I sat just behind him with Mangkhara and Ouanna. At the end of the concert, which he told me he enjoyed very much, and I don't think he was being merely polite, I presented the musicians to him.

Last evening we held a gala Vientiane concert for the benefit of the Red Cross. Moune, as you know, is president of the Women's Red Cross of Laos. She works hard at it, and was pleased that this fund-raising event was being held. This was under the sponsorship of the prime minister and, unlike the other Lloyd concerts, had a distinguished, dressy audience which included Prince and Princess Souvanna Phouma, many ambassadors, and representatives of the Soviet Union. We had borrowed some psychedelic lighting from the Third Eye bar, and this made for fascinating stage effects. Moune and I had wondered whether her father, no fan of jazz, would stay through the performance, but he did and met with the musicians afterward.

This program gave me a feeling of enormous satisfaction, similar to what I had felt after some of those programs in France. I drafted a cable to the State Department to commend them on their choice of Charles Lloyd for Laos.

———

Prince Souvanna while addressing the National Assembly on Friday reiterated that the North Vietnamese were continuing their military activities against the Lao government. There was nothing new in that statement. This is common knowledge, and any observer of the Lao scene would concur.

Today, however, the Ministry of Foreign Affairs in Hanoi savagely denounced the prime minister and called his charges slanderous. The North Vietnamese declared that the problem was American intervention and aggression—and sabotage by the United States of the Geneva accords.

A barefaced lie violates all our codes of rationality, let alone ethics. How to react? If you shout "Liar!" you know that the one capable of pronouncing the lie is going to brush off the accusation.

The historical big lie is all too common in our times. And here it is again, directed against the little kingdom.

Princess Souvanna left yesterday for Paris. We went to the airport to see her off, as did a good many others, diplomats and Lao. In the evening, Moune and I had dinner with her father, just the three of us. At such moments, I feel a certain guilt in the realization that I shall be responsible for placing a great geographical distance between this devoted father and daughter.

Moune, if she were to remain in the Lao Ministry of Foreign Affairs, would soon become an ambassador. And she would be excellent in that role. Perhaps I should resign from the American Foreign Service in order to become the ambassador's spouse. An amusing idea, but a fleeting one that will receive no further consideration.

These last weeks, while Moune has supposedly been regaining her vitality, she has been occupied with her work at the Ministry, busy with her responsibilities at the Red Cross, attentive to her father's affairs, and adding elegant finishing touches to the ranch house. We have been going out evening after evening, often dancing, with Moune in appearance a very pretty young lady without a serious thought. During these same weeks, she, at the behest of the government, and with the strong encouragement of Western ambassadors, wrote and organized an important document, a *White Book on the Violations of the 1962 Geneva Accords by the Government of North Vietnam*. It has just been published.

In the introduction, Prince Souvanna declares that North Vietnamese aggression against Laos is indisputable and that the ambition of the Hanoi government is to have the kingdom become a satellite to serve as an eventual base for other North Vietnamese conquests. He states that the unique ambition of the Lao people is to have peace.

Moune, in the text proper, tells how despite its signature of the accords of Geneva to respect and guarantee the neutrality and sovereignty of the Kingdom of Laos, the North Vietnamese have intensified their war against Laos. She writes that the Lao government has long known that it is confronted by a foreign aggressor and not by a rebel political party, as the Pathet Lao and North Vietnamese pretend.

The main body of the book presents in some detail attacks against Laos in recent years. It includes interviews with captured North Vietnamese prisoners of war and contains many photos of people, areas, and captured arms that substantiate the text.

In her conclusions, Moune comments that some have accused the kingdom of collusion with the United States. She answers the charge first by citing Article 6 of the Geneva Accords: the introduction of war materials into Laos is prohibited *except* for arms which the government of Laos deems necessary for its defense, and then by explaining that in this latter instance, faced with the urgent need for defense weapons, the kingdom requested them from America.

This new *White Book* is being well received. Bill Sullivan mentioned that it will be of real value in presenting the case of Laos at international gatherings.

Last December, people remarked how poor relations were between the French and American communities in this city. Nevertheless, and perhaps because I came here from France, I was wonderfully well received by the French, including the ambassador and his wife.

Now I am attempting some programming to improve the relations. Georges Marguier, the French cultural attaché, is an art historian. I have arranged for him to give an illustrated lecture in French for a predominantly French audience on contemporary American art, and the talk will be under American sponsorship. We are not apt to attract a large audience, but baby steps precede giant steps.

Moune has written to Governor Harriman to thank him for keeping the situation in Laos firmly on the agenda of the Vietnamese talks now taking place in Paris. We are very happy that it is he who is the American spokesman at these sessions.

And since she was writing to him, she took him into her confidence and told him what we are not yet able to announce: we are getting married.

Prince Souvanna has been up to Luang Prabang for several days. He enjoys time spent in that magnificent town, and I think he prefers it to Vientiane, although his relations with his cousin, the king, are, I gather, sometimes strained. He has an old family house in LP, but last evening he spoke to us about his plans to build another home there, one in which he eventually hopes to retire. He was trained in France as an architect, and when he can, which is infrequently, he reverts to that profession. I have watched him sketch houses and buildings, and he takes a keen interest in whatever is being constructed for the government.

He is leaving for France later this week for his annual summer visit to the quiet spa of Plombières-les-Bains in the Vosges Mountains. There he can relax and regain the physical strength needed for the leadership of the little kingdom.

At dinner last evening, just the three of us, we naturally got onto the topic of the American political campaign. It was the election of Kennedy and the choice of Governor Harriman as his envoy to Asia that changed the course of Lao history, and the prince is devoted to the governor for what he has done on behalf of the kingdom. In this next election, the prince wonders what the American attitude toward Laos will be if Richard Nixon becomes president. That possibility seems to trouble him, especially since Nixon had been vice president in an administration hostile to Souvanna. The idea of Nixon as president bothers me, too, for some of the same and other reasons.

You probably read in *The New York Times* the story on the press conference which Moune's father held in Paris. His statement that the United States should not stop its bombing of North Vietnam until that country withdraws its 40,000 soldiers from Laos was accompanied by the explanation that there can be no peace in the region as long as those Vietnamese troops are present. True enough, but I was surprised that he made such a statement, and even more surprised that he did so publicly. Notwithstanding Hanoi's war against the little kingdom and the harassment the prime minister accordingly suffers, Souvanna is a man of peace and not of war.

I was amused by the interviewer's description of him: "square jawed and quiet voiced . . . comfortably seated in an overstuffed armchair." The prince receives more attention for his undramatic manner than most national leaders can hope to obtain by ranting and histrionics.

Social life in Vientiane's diplomatic circle often takes unusual turns, and sometimes these seem sort of silly. Moune and I are friendly with the chief commissioner of the International Control Commission, an Indian, and we appreciate his attempts to offset the Polish commissioner's constant efforts to block any investigations of communist activities. The chief is hosting a dinner next week, a purely protocol affair, in honor of the Soviet ambassador, and has invited us to be among his guests. This is silly, but the explanation surely is that he wants to have Moune present and has decided the best way to arrange that is to invite me as well.

Yesterday, at the Lao Embassy in Paris, Prince Souvanna gave a press conference during which he surprised the press and pleased me. Only four weeks ago, when he arrived in Paris, he had during another press conference called for the continued bombing of North Vietnam until Hanoi removes its troops from Laos. Yesterday he declared that in the interim the Pathet Lao–North Vietnamese military actions have markedly diminished and that therefore the United States should discontinue the bombing.

There has been a notable lull in the fighting in recent weeks, perhaps as a result of the ongoing talks in Paris. Whatever the reason, I hope the president does call off the bombing raids. Hanoi may be playing yet another move in its game of deception, but this could present a possible breakthrough in the war. By heeding Souvanna's advice, we have little to lose, and, although unlikely, peace might be gained.

Some are suggesting that the prince's latest remarks may have been influenced by his private conversations with President de Gaulle on the previous day. I doubt that. De Gaulle and Souvanna admire each other, but Moune's father pronounces only his own convictions.

◆ ◆ ◆

August, September 1968

If the Kingdom of Laos has a guardian angel in the Western world, he is surely Averell Harriman. Yesterday in Paris, the governor not only went on at length about the North Vietnamese violations of the Geneva accords on Laos but then invited the head of the Hanoi delegation to go to Laos with him in order to observe first hand the evidences of North Vietnamese aggression against the kingdom. That's our governor!

———————

Should the little kingdom ever become a tourist attraction, the tourist season would have to be the winter. The frequent downpours of the summer turn the earth into mud and make life in the city a dashing in-and-out between torrential—and I am accurately employing that overused adjective—showers. In the dry season, one frequently entertains on the lawns. Now, in the wet season, one can never be certain that the garden will be receptive to receptions.

Prince Souvanna returned from France in what seems to be relatively good health but with somewhat troubled spirits. The Paris talks on Vietnam are not progressing, and although the military activities in this country have somewhat abated, when the wet season ends they will surely be renewed.

Also, it has not helped the prince's morale to learn that one of his nephews, Prince Ariya, a son of Prince Souphanouvong, has been killed. According to the report we've received, the circumstances are mysterious. The murder is said to have taken place months ago in Samneua, Pathet Lao territory in the north, where Ariya was vacationing after he had received a degree in engineering from the University of Moscow. The report says that Ariya was stabbed to death, but why and by whom we do not know.

This brings to mind the relationship between the two half-brothers, Souvanna and Souphanouvong. Here they are, the leaders of two warring factions. Souvanna often denounces Souphanouvong's Pathet Lao, and the Hanoi government, whose troops are in this country under the pretext of being Pathet Lao soldiers, makes vehement charges against the prime minister.

Despite this, a family closeness continues to exist. Moune's mother believes Souphanouvong has always been jealous of his elder half-brother. But Souvanna, while deploring and condemning Souphanouvong's political and military deeds, apparently has never fully lost his affection for him.

Souphanouvong has many children, but who can tell how deeply this loss of a son may affect him? What we can be sure of is it will not alter Souphanouvong's ambitions to overthrow his brother and transform the kingdom into a vassal of the North Vietnamese.

Worried about the future of this kingdom, I read the reports from home and become equally worried about what is happening in our own country. I did not want Hubert Humphrey to be the candidate. All of my recent negative reactions toward him have been forcefully strengthened by what took place at the Chicago convention, his acceptance speech, and his defense of Mayor Daley. I have no illusions about Richard Nixon—I could never have confidence in him—but I wonder if he, as president, might not be more effective in resolving the Southeast Asia situation than Humphrey could be. Of the four candidates, the only one I like is Muskie. I wish he were going to be president.

Dan Oleksiw, the Information Agency's director for Asia, was here for the weekend, and the senior officers of the post were involved with him in long discussions about our operation. Dan is a good man, enormous physically and with a keen mind. I gather that he intimidates some of the agency, and it's easy to see why. Alone with me for a moment, he told me he was looking forward to meeting Moune on Sunday. Keith Adamson, our new public affairs officer, had scheduled Dan for breakfast at the ranch house that day.

On Saturday evening, Dan was a guest of honor at a large reception Ambassador Sullivan gave at his residence. Moune and I were invited to it and also to a black tie dinner at the French ambassador's residence, and the schedule was such that we had to go directly from one to the other. Consequently, we arrived at our ambassador's conspicuously in formal clothes. Moune was wearing a magnificent white silk gown with brocaded red roses, and she looked radiant. It was there that Dan met her and conversed with her far longer than mere politeness demanded. He is obviously happy to welcome her as the wife of an agency officer.

Sunday morning, Dan and Keith joined us at home for Bloody Marys, eggs, and such. Dan told us that he had discussed with the ambassador our situation, and they agreed that my request to leave soon after the wedding was the correct decision. I am growing too sensitive in my position. I was angry recently when the new deputy public affairs officer, who incidentally is supposed to be the officer to whom I report, said that since I spent so much time with the prime minister it would be helpful if I let them know more of his reactions on different issues. This DPAO is a fool, and Bill Sullivan would never make such a suggestion, but there it was—spelled out. Besides that, Laos guards its neutrality, and my regular presence in the prime minister's house could be a cause of embarrassment. And finally, for Moune, too, there are just too many demands made upon her here.

So we will be leaving Laos. Dan could not say at this time what my new assignment will be, but he knows we would love to be posted in Europe.

As for the dinner at the French embassy, it was a dull affair saved by the after-dinner bridge, where I was fortunate enough to be at the prince's table.

Before one arrives at the bamboo-lined private road that leads to the ranch house, one has to traverse a public road that the rainy season has been unkind to. Large potholes make it risky. Since we entertain a good deal and some of our guests are distinguished, something has to be done about the road. At home one would complain to the department of roads and hope that repairs would be undertaken. Here that routine is apt to prove ineffective. There is not much sense of urgency among the bureaucrats.

So I did something I shouldn't have done. I committed an abuse of privilege. Ngon Sananikone, the minister of works and transportation, is an old friend and has been a visitor to our house. I telephoned and asked if I could see him. He promptly suggested I stop by his house late that morning. I did so, he quickly assured me that the road would be repaired, and then drinks were served.

Ngon encapsulates many of the most delightful Lao characteristics. He is essentially a jovial man with a pudgy frame and a round smiling face. He exudes humor and warmth. He is also an astute political figure. Ngon is often mentioned as a potential prime minister and actually has long been a rival of Souvanna.

My call on him did not end with drinks. Two members of his family joined us, then he insisted I telephone Moune and have her lunch with us at the Hotel Lan Xang, where we went on for too long with food and wines and Ngon recounting his funny, sometimes ribald stories. The Lao find rich humor in almost everything.

I didn't want to ask a favor of Ngon, but I did. I don't agree with his politics, but I do enjoy his company.

Early yesterday morning I was working at my desk when Moune telephoned from her office to say she wanted to see me, so I hopped into the little car and raced over to the ministry. A cable had arrived from her lawyer in Paris containing the news we have been awaiting. The necessary papers for Moune's divorce should be on their way from France within a week or two, and then we shall be married as soon as possible. I wonder if two people were ever more eager to be united in matrimony.

We had dinner with her father in the evening. I spoke to him again about my regret at taking Moune away from him. Even Bill

Sullivan expressed concern about this. But the prince repeated that Moune's happiness was of primary importance to him. If her leaving did create problems, we would stay even though that would mean my retiring from the service.

He also told us he had decided to move into the fascinating house the government is building along the Mekong, not far from the ranch house. Here we have an example of the prince as architect, for he designed this most unusual concept. There are two wings connected by attractive covered walkways. The larger, more imposing, wing is for representational purposes. It contains a fine entrance hall, a good office, a huge salon, and a dining room which can readily seat fifty persons. The long wall of the dining room opens onto an ever larger terrace, with trees, that overlooks the river, so that the outside flows in unobstructed. This wing is grand but not ostentatious. The lines are clean-cut but not box-like and are punctuated by interesting angles.

The other wing is for family purposes. The dining room, kitchen, and servants' quarters are on the first floor, and upstairs are the living room with its balcony on the river and four large bedrooms, each with its own bathroom. Overall this is an ingenious, handsome, and extremely practical arrangement. It permits the prime minister to perform his official and representational duties at home and still be able to live in a separate family environment immediately at hand.

———————

Eugene Black, the distinguished former head of the International Bank for Reconstruction and Development, is here for a few days. He was met at the airport by the prime minister, who is having a dinner for him this evening.

Black has been discussing the extraordinary Pa Mong project. Work on it began some years ago. Its principal objective is to build a huge dam just north of Vientiane which will provide countries in this area with far, far more energy than they now possess. Thailand, Laos, Cambodia, and South Vietnam would be beneficiaries. The Mekong Project, as it is popularly known, has a marvelous potential. If only these countries were not at war!

But the real reason for Black's presence is as an envoy of

President Johnson, to assure these countries that despite the uproar at home and demands that the United States pull out of Southeast Asia, we will not pull out, no matter who the president will be, Black says. From what we gather, in the various countries in which he has recently been to make this pitch—the Philippines, Cambodia, Taiwan, Japan, and Thailand—his assurances are being greeted with a certain skepticism. This skepticism is all too comprehensive.

We spent the last two days of the month in Chiang Mai, a very special city for us. John and Pat Ryan, the Australian ambassador and his wife, had to touch down on several posts in Laos and then across the river in Thailand. They invited us to join them abroad the Australian army aircraft.

One of our brief stops was at Ban Houey Sai, a green, hilly town north of here on the Mekong. Each time I visit it, I climb the hill to what had once been a French Foreign Legion port. A tarnished plaque continues to proclaim what it once was and no longer is, and there are remnants of the stone walls. I like to stand among the ruins, look down on the broad river below, and try to imagine what life was like for legionnaires. The site is lovely, and to have been posted in Laos those many years ago should I have been more agreeable than rigorous.

In Chiang Mai, Moune and I must look just foolish. We have such a sentimental attachment to that city we do little other than walk about and smile and smile and smile.

Although Prince Souvanna agreed to the American bombing of that remote area of Laos through which the Ho Chi Minh Trail and the North Vietnamese supplies pass, the prince has refused to allow American troops back in the kingdom ever since they departed in 1962, in accordance with the Geneva agreements. This resolution on his part seems to me so right, so absolutely necessary, that I have imagined it would be almost universally understood. How wrong I was.

Over drinks at the bar of the Lan Xang Hotel the other afternoon, someone from the American army attaché's office, someone who had perhaps consumed more alcohol than he could tolerate, told me that General Westmoreland was getting frustrated with the way the war was going in Vietnam. Therefore, the general had decided that he needed a friendlier, less neutral government in the little kingdom, one that would welcome back the American soldiers. I said nothing in reply but was profoundly shaken.

After mulling it over for two days, I asked to see Ambassador Sullivan. In his office I repeated the rumor I had heard. Bill Sullivan looked at me for a moment and then, neither denying nor affirming the rumor, said: "As long as I am ambassador here, the American government will fully support the government of Souvanna Phouma."

I know that Bill Sullivan meant precisely what he said, and I am greatful that he is our ambassador. But I also believe that General Westmoreland would like to overthrow the government of Laos. And I pity our country that has placed such a man in his position of leadership.

◆ ◆ ◆

October, November 1968

We spent most of the weekend moving the prime minister into his new residence. Fortunately he was up in Luang Prabang, which allowed us a freer hand. We had the two lavish crystal chandeliers from the living room of the old residence rehung in the new dining room. This gives what was already a handsome room a European elegance. And we gathered together the prince's collection of oil paintings and arranged them all on the far side of the salon: they add much interest to the room. Then we wondered what the prince's reaction would be, but when he returned home he looked at the paintings and said nothing, which means approval of a sort.

Moune likes wallpapers and is determined to use them in the entrance hall and bathrooms. Since wallpaper seems never to have been used in this country and no one could be found to work in this medium, she, family and friends, including the wives of the French,

Thai, and Australian ambassadors, may be found at odd moments perched on the tops of ladders juggling rolls of paper and pots of glue. I made an effort to help but was dismissed as being too clumsy.

Thank heavens. What we have been waiting for from Paris has arrived, and Moune is free to marry. We wanted to have a small ceremony this weekend, but her father informed us that weddings are not held in Laos when the moon is declining. The Buddhists, not unlike the Jews, make much of the new moon. He asked that the wedding wait until the twenty-first of this month and added that he would like it to be a *baci* held at his home. A *baci* is a Lao rite held for arrivals, departures, marriages, and births. After writing the above sentences, I reached up on the bookshelves and took down an essay by my old friend, Nhouy Abhay.

He writes, "The *baci* is the Lao ceremony par excellence, the one with which this kind people expresses its *joie de vivre* and warmheartedness. Whether magnificent or modest, grave or familiar but always ardent and sincere, the *baci* is an expression of welcome. It is a smile to life, a forgiveness of trespasses and unshakable confidence in the supreme powers of the gods and the Buddha."

Despite Nhouy's definition, the *baci* is not a religious ceremony per se, for the prayers are conducted not by a monk but by a venerable elder. Anyway, since we will be married with a *baci*, we will be inviting not only family but a few friends as well. However, Moune and I are determined to keep the invitation list short.

The date for the big event has been changed again. This is now a comedy of sorts. As of today, but subject to further modifications, the wedding is scheduled for this coming Tuesday, the twenty-second, in the afternoon.

In the meantime, Moune continues to run a section of her ministry and the Red Cross, and serves as decorator for her father's new residence. And we both wait for word from Washington as to where we go from here. Although we have made no announcements, news about us is spreading, and I've received several letters of congratulations from friends in the States and in Europe.

There was a formal Red Cross benefit last night, and Moune not only arranged all of the details for the entire affair but then presided gorgeously in a Lao costume.

Saturday was Prince Souvanna's birthday. A dozen *bonzes* came in the morning to bless the house. At the end of the afternoon, some two hundred persons came to wish the prince happiness, to inspect the house and terrace, and to drink champagne. When the crowd was at its greatest, all of the lights went out, not by design but because of a circuit failure. Many candles were quickly lit, which gave the house and terrace an enchanting glow.

Rumor has it that we will be going to Washington as our next posting. Someone in personnel is refusing to allow me a direct transfer by arguing that because I am marrying an alien we must put in time in the States. To tell that personnel man that my alien already knows America and was a student for a year at Harvard is not apt to satisfy the cravings of a bureaucrat.

A fresh-out-of-Harvard stringer for *Time* magazine is in Vientiane on his first job and trying to gain a reputation. His name is Timothy Allman. He is extremely bright, and we think he may in time become a well-known journalist. Today was his birthday, and Moune invited him to the ranch house for lunch. Beneath that aggressive facade all news gatherers must possess, he seems to have a pleasing shyness.

Peter and Marian Edelman are visiting Vientiane. Peter had been one of Robert Kennedy's legal assistants and before that, Arthur Goldberg's law clerk. Marian was the brave legal counsel for the

NAACP in Mississippi. Bill Sullivan's weekend calendar was completely booked, and so he asked us if we could entertain the Edelmans on Friday evening, which we were delighted to do. They are an impressive couple and are making penetrating observations on their visit to Asia. Perhaps because they know how to ask pertinent questions.

We're getting married in three days and changing plans about a so-called honeymoon. We have not yet heard from Washington about our future destination, and my father-in-law is holding a large dinner on Thursday for a visiting Thai dignitary at which Moune thinks she should be present. But in truth, we don't need a formal honeymoon.

We ordered our wedding announcements. They are simple and state in French that Moune S. P. and P. J. S. are happy to announce their marriage in Vientiane on October 22. I thought that Moune might wish to use her title, but she said no. I should have known that a true princess does not announce herself.

By the way, according to Asian custom, a princess does not lose her title when she marries a commoner. A commoner! Is that what I've become? I never thought of myself as that.

Our only regret yesterday was that you were not with us. Otherwise it was exactly as we wished it to be.

In the morning we freed dozens of little birds from their cages and watched them fly away. Then we took dozens of little fish in buckets and emptied the buckets into the Mekong and watched them swim away. Alongside the family wing of father's new residence, we planted two banana trees close to each other.

As for the wedding itself, let me try to describe it as you would have experienced it.

As you enter the main wing of the house, you leave your shoes in the hall and then proceed into the salon, where the floor has been covered by rugs. Some thirty friends are there, sitting in close proximity to each other to give a sense of unity to the gathering.

Toward the far side of the room is a large platter on which is a tall silver bowl from which rise thin bamboo sticks, each entwined with flowers. The flowers are the focal point, for the *baci* is a floral offering. From the flowers on the bamboo sticks, thin pieces of cotton thread hang—they will be used later. Also on the platter are banana leaves cupped and filled with flowers, small bottles of alcohol, hard-boiled eggs, rice and small rice cakes, and silver candlesticks in which candles burn. This platter will surely remind you of the Passover seder table. The fragrance in the room is burning incense.

After the guests are seated on the rugs and the venerable old man who will officiate has placed himself behind the platter, Prince Souvanna Phouma enters. He is in a white Lao jacket, and he sits in front of the silver bowl of flowers. Moune comes into the room. She is in a traditional gold-encrusted mauve silk costume, her hair in a high topknot around which is tied a gold chain. She sits on the rug next to her father. Finally I, suddenly very nervous, enter the room. I'm wearing a dark blue summer Brooks Brothers suit. I sit on the other side of the prince.

As the old man starts to intone his prayers, all of us in the room bring the palms of our hands together and rest our foreheads on the tops of our fingers. The prayers are addressed to the spirits that should reside within the body but have fled. Nhouy has translated them this way:

> Come back, oh soul, come along the path which has been
>   cleansed and is now open to you;
> Come home;
> Wade through the river if it only comes up to your chest;
> Swim if the river is deep;
> When you arrive at the light don't hide in the huts;
> When you come up to the tree stump, do not rest you
>   head upon it.
> Do not fear when you come near;
> Have no fear of ghosts or geniuses. . . .
> Come back this day, oh soul who has gone to a new birth
>   in the uninhabited village, where live the twin-tail
>   snakes, and where reign the goddesses with two knots
>   of hair;

Do not linger on the way, neither with the *Phis* [spirits] or
in the mountains;
Come home to your home made of smooth planks,
covered with thick hay and of which the foundation
· piles and the timber of its framework have been pulled
by the mighty elephants;
Come back to this stately abode where you shall not be
short of anything, where you shall not be ill-treated
either by your uncles or your parents, where all will
love you as gold and cherish you as a precious stone;
Come back, stand before this platter, and stay home from
now on!

Then the old man wishes us the universal wishes: long life,
health, happiness, freedom from want, and strength. "Be as strong
as the antlers of a stag, as the jaws of a wild bear or as the tusks of
an elephant."

At this time, those in the room who wish make their way
forward, on their knees if they can, until they reach the silver bowl,
from which they take the hanging strings and tie them about the
wrists of Moune and myself. These strings bind our souls within
our bodies. As the string tying takes place, the others stretch their
hands to touch the person in front of them so that everyone may
take part in this blessing.

The *baci* over, we went into the dining room, cut the handsome
wedding cake, and drank champagne. Then Moune and I went
back to the ranch house and opened another bottle of champagne,
which we drank with our dear servants, Ky and Mien. Later the
two of us had a fine dinner, which Mien had prepared.

And so, my dear sister and brother, I am no longer a bachelor
but very much a married man.

———————

The peace talks in Paris, after these many months, seem to be
reaching a possible breakthrough and an answer to the question:
Will we or will we not continue to bomb North Vietnam? Here in
Vientiane, there is every reason to favor whatever action is taken
against the North Vietnamese, for they continue to wage an

undeclared war against Laos. Despite that, for many of the influential Lao, the ongoing bombing is appalling. Their Buddhist upbringing abhors killing.

My father-in-law has devoted himself to his country and its independence, and now his earlier successes are being undermined and threatened by Hanoi. In July he had declared himself in favor of the American bombing with conditions, but within weeks, in another public statement, he expressed the hope that the bombing would desist. He has made no further public statement on the matter and, I suspect, is unlikely to make any.

I don't know that this proves anything except perhaps that no matter how vile the enemy, to conduct a defensive war is natural and instinctive, but to support an offensive war requires a type of mentality alien to the gentle people of the little kingdom.

His Majesty held his annual reception for the diplomats last evening at his Vientiane palace. The spacious grounds sweep down to the river and were especially beautiful in the light of the flickering lamps. Late in the evening, when all went to their seats to watch the exquisite classical dancers, I parted from the diplomats to take a place with my new family. This gave my father-in-law the occasion to present me to the king. I had been presented to the king at several official functions, but this time, of course, was different. He wears a kind but quizzical expression, and there is a unique yet sympathetic air about him. Prince Souvanna seemed pleased when he presented me, and Moune was by my side in a low, graceful reverence before His Majesty.

Moune and I invited some thirty members of the family to the ranch house for dinner, and that very afternoon, to our great pleasure, Princess Souvanna returned from Paris and was able to join us.

My wife/decorator hastened about with final preparations and gave the little house a charming air, with tables set on the lawn. The family was a delightful group. My mother-in-law, Moune, and I changed tables with each course, so that we managed to spend time with each of our guests. Some I had hardly met, but I had no difficulty in addressing them. Each could be called *Altesse*.

I was unhappy today to learn that I had been set for a vacant slot in the cultural affairs section of our embassy in London, but good friends in Washington—Dan Oleksiw and Dave Shepperd among them— had convinced personnel that it would be wasteful to send me to London instead of to a French-speaking country. How we would have enjoyed a few years in London! And now, with time approaching for our departure, we still don't know where we are going.

Definite word: my replacement arrives in two weeks, and so we must leave although uncertain as to where. We have set the evening of November 29 as the date for a large farewell party the prince and princess wish to hold for us at their residence. Our wedding had been an intimate affair; this party will be for more than a hundred persons.

And so, as expected, Richard Nixon is to be our next president. Given the bellicose nature of the North Vietnamese, it will be extraordinarily difficult to bring this war to a halt without sacrificing South Vietnam or my beloved Laos, but let us fervently hope that he will find a way to achieve this.

I am not sorry that Humphrey lost.

My new assignment arrived: consul and branch public affairs officer in Marseille. I will be engaged in the same type of programming I did out of Paris, but this time, I shall live in Provence and shall be exclusively occupied with the area from Monaco to Bordeaux. Was there ever such a glorious assignment? Moune and I couldn't be happier. How fortunate we are!

We have to be in Paris for staff meetings on Monday, December 2, so we shall leave here on Saturday, the thirtieth, after our large farewell party, and arrive in Paris on Sunday morning. We will have to find time to pack, since we are involved daily with lunches and dinners of adieu.

Last evening was exceptional. Sisouk na Champassak and Christiane held a small and elegant dinner for us with the British and Japanese ambassadors and their wives among the guests.

Sisouk apparently was always a man of great potential. His intelligence, determination, courage, and general attractiveness stood him in excellent stead when he was the Lao ambassador to the United Nations. A nephew of Prince Boun Oum, he was by formation a staunch rightist, at one time even an ally of Phoumi Nosavan. But now Sisouk devotes all of his enormous abilities to the ardent support of Prince Souvanna's government and policies.

No wonder that with such leadership the neutralist government survives against great odds.

The little kingdom militarily and economically has, as everyone knows, gargantuan problems, but life goes on in fine style, and I like it this way. Last evening Le Bal des Fleurs, a large charity dance, was held under the patronage of the crown prince at the Lan Xang Hotel. We were invited to the Sullivan's for a dinner party before the ball, and then we all went off to an evening of music and dancing and champagne. I repeat: I like this style, especially since none of us has illusions. We recognize its ephemerality.

We arrived in Paris yesterday, and even in the gray of winter, with its buildings and monuments obscured by the bleak, thick weather, this city is a joy to see and be in.

For our last evening in Vientiane, some hundred and fifty persons in evening dress came to the prime minister's residence, were welcomed by Princess Souvanna, Moune, Panya, and myself, then proceeded out onto the terrace, where they strolled on the bank of the Mekong and admired the low-hanging moon, sat at small lamp-lit tables, danced the *lam vong* and other dances played by the best musicians in the country, ate a midnight supper, joined the prince in a champagne toast, and remained for hours, with many commenting that this had been the most beautiful of parties.

The next day at the airport, in Vientiane fashion, a crowd of friends was there to see us off. It was terribly sad to leave the little kingdom, but, although I may not look it, I am now half Lao and shall be returning.

V

Kingdom Gone

1969–1984

On rereading my letters from Vientiane, I realize that my personal happiness, which was intricately involved with Laos and which could hardly have been greater, obscures what lay just beneath the surface: a desperate fear of what was happening to the little kingdom. And when Moune and I departed for France, that fear naturally remained with us.

❊ ❊ ❊

The North Vietnamese expansion continued.

1969: The North Vietnamese overran the Lao army at Muong Sai in June. That autumn, the People's Republic of China completed the construction of a road leading directly into northern Laos, an event applauded by those who hoped that China's presence in the country might help keep a check on Hanoi.

1970: Six thousand North Vietnamese soldiers captured the Plain of Jars and then went on to take the important towns of Attopeu and Saravane. In subsequent years, the two towns were retaken by the government.

1971: In May, North Vietnamese soldiers seized the towns of Paksong and Dong Hene, thereby posing a threat to the vital Mekong Valley cities of Savannakhet and Pakse. The Lao army regained Paksong in September, but lost eleven hundred men doing so. In late December, the North Vietnamese took back Paksong and the Bolovens Plateau.

1972: As the North Vietnamese army continued its advance, many thousands of civilians fled from the town of Long Tien and its environs, increasing heavily the number of refugees who already made up more than one fourth of the population.

1973: Saravane was again captured by the invading army.

◆ ◆ ◆

It troubled me to hear how often, particularly in America, when Laos was mentioned, it would be discussed—and dismissed—as simply another Indochinese nation. Laos was very different from the others. Its tripartite government came into existence with the most eminent of midwives, England, France and the United States among the Western powers, the Soviet Union, the People's Republic of China, and North Vietnam among the communist sponsors.

There could be no question then about the absolute legitimacy of this little country, nor of its prime minister, Prince Souvanna Phouma, the choice of the fourteen nations at Geneva.

The little kingdom was distinctive in many ways. Although corruption had been rife under Phoumi Nosavan, Laos was remarkably free of financial scandal from the time of the establishment of the tripartite government and Souvanna's appointment of Sisouk na Champassak as minister of finance. Once in Paris, Princess Souvanna Phouma remarked to me with an expression which managed amusingly to combine a certain regret with genuine admiration that my father-in-law was the rare head of government who had not taken advantage of his position to enrich himself.

❊ ❊ ❊

Souvanna Phouma never ceased to urge the Pathet Lao to return to the government and to occupy the ministerial posts he kept open for them. Until the end, he tried to abide by the Geneva accords. In 1971, South Vietnamese soldiers crossed the border into Laos to fight against the North Vietnamese soldiers in the vicinity of the Ho Chi Minh Trail. Even though this was undertaken to fight against the enemies of Laos, the prince decried the action, declared he had not been consulted in the matter, and demanded that the Geneva accords be respected by others even if flauntingly violated by Hanoi. (President Nixon, however, stated that the South Vietnamese army drive into Laos had improved the overall situation.)

The little kingdom struggled valiantly for its neutrality—and its survival.

◆ ◆ ◆

A sprawling house in a spacious park overlooking the Mediterranean offered to us by the State Department was our home in Marseille in 1969 and 1970. I particularly remember the wall of French doors which opened from the salon onto a sweeping lawn suspended above the sea. Our arrival coincided with that of the new consul general, Philip Chadbourn, my colleague during the Paris meeting of the three princes of Laos. Faithful Gabrielle agreed to leave for a while her beloved Paris to be our cook and housekeeper. My principal task was the establishment of relations with newspaper publishers and editors to provide them with American informational materials, with museum directors to offer them American exhibitions, and with university rectors and faculty members to further the exchange of programs and people between French and American universities. Across southern France I traveled, from Monte Carlo to Bordeaux, and Moune went with me.

Sometimes there were meetings to attend in Paris. We would generally drive up and reach Moune's Paris apartment in the evening. On one such occasion, her mother who lived nearby, telephoned in the morning to welcome us and I had to inform her that her daughter was in bed and feeling not at all well. An hour later I gained new insight into the Princess Souvanna Phouma. She arrived at our door with a container of rice in chicken broth which she had just prepared. I laughed at the revelation that beneath the exterior of this *grand dame* lurked a Jewish mama.

Moune and I would spend a few days with her father during his summer fortnight at Plombières in the Vosges Mountains. It was here in the middle of the last century that Napolean III met with Cavour to design a unified Italy, and the town seems in many ways to have remained in the nineteenth century. On our very first evening there, Moune and I strolled about the quiet village and saw light gleaming through the stained glass windows of the old church that dominated the landscape. We approached; angelic music came from within. We entered; a Baroque concert was being performed. This town permitted Prince Souvanna Phouma to unwind from the tensions that were with him elsewhere. Here he enjoyed his daily hour at the spa, books, paths to roam, games of bridge, and a good choice of half-day auto excursions, including one to that architectural masterpiece, Le Corbusier's church at Ronchamp.

There had been times in the past when the prince had considered exiling himself from Laos, most notably when American forces had actively supported Phoumi Nosavan's rebellion. But by 1969 any thought of his ever leaving his own country had disappeared. Now the Lao people, excluding the communists but including the rightists who had opposed him for all of those years, were united behind him. If, as our problems in Vietnam grew ever graver, American interest in Laos had started to fade and American material support lessened, the United States and the Western nations clearly approved of him and morally supported him.

Souvanna was a realist. His efforts for—his dreams of—a Laos that would be an independent, neutralist, democratically governed monarchy were, he knew, unlikely to be realized, but he continued in his diplomatic and political endeavors to act as though that desired future were attainable. Expert bridge players upon being dealt a poor hand play it as though the contract could succeed.

◆ ◆ ◆

Washington was the next assignment, and in 1971 I was given the position of cultural coordinator for Western Europe at the United States Information Agency. The title was more impressive than the actual duties it entailed.

Moune and I purchased a home. We did not find what we wanted or could afford until dear friends, Richard and Christine Coe, offered to sell us a 150-year-old house in Georgetown. It had fireplaces in the living room, dining room, and study, a small walled garden, and a graceful open staircase that made a complete turn as it climbed from the sitting room to the upstairs bedrooms. We looked at the staircase, immediately bought the house, and never regretted it.

When my father-in-law was in Washington on an official visit, he came to the house for dinner. What was in those days a quiet neighborhood was somewhat disrupted by this event, for too many Secret Service agents were too much in evidence. The house even had to submit to an inspection before the prince was permitted to enter.

During this period, the Lao ambassador to the United States was Prince Khammao, a brother of the king, and his wife was Princess Khamla, a full sister of Moune's father. I first met them when Moune and I were briefly in London at the time Khammao was Lao ambassador to the Court of Saint James. In Washington we saw them frequently, and I became very fond of them. Khammao was a quiet man who loved fishing, while Khamla was an extremely intelligent woman of great energy. They treated me as a close member of the family, and when Moune had to go to Paris for several weeks, they insisted that I dine with them as regularly as I would have had Moune been there.

One Sunday evening, Moune and I went to the Lao embassy and found Prince Khammao definitely morose. Alone with him, I asked what was troubling him, and he told me. A resolution before the United Nations was being supported by almost all of the Third World nations and opposed by the United States. Laos was in favor of the resolution. That Sunday afternoon, Prince Khammao had been summoned to the State Department for an "emergency meeting" with the assistant secretary for Asian affairs. According to the prince, the assistant secretary had demanded that Laos change its intended vote. Khammao was reminded of how indebted the little kingdom was to America, and the threat was made that we would no longer hold such a friendly attitude if Laos failed to vote with us on this question. It must have been a nasty session, although I suspect that quiet Khammao said little as he refused to accept the arrogant demands made upon him and his country. The prince informed me that he had no intention of being spoken to in this manner and that he was going to ask to be replaced as ambassador to Washington.

This incident is certainly not typical of the relations between the United States and Laos, but it did happen, should not have happened, and suggests some of the difficulties that might ensue in the relationship of a small country vis-à-vis a great power, especially when a high-ranking official within the power structure lacks basic respect for those with whom he is dealing. And the members of the royal Lao family were clothed in enormous dignity.

Our house was just down the street from that of the great American benefactor of the little kingdom, Averell Harriman, and we enjoyed occasional visits with the governor and his lovely wife Pamela.

After two years, we were eager to move on to another overseas post, and several possibilities were in the offing. One morning I called on the personnel officer responsible for finding my new assignment, and he informed me that word had just been received that the position of cultural attaché in Bangkok was unexpectedly opening within the year. I remember literally jumping out of my seat and exclaiming: "That's for me. Don't offer it to anyone else." I could not serve again in Laos, but being in Bangkok would be the closest alternative.

The personnel officer, after gaining the necessary approval

from the bureaucracy, sent a cable requesting acceptance of my appointment from our embassy in Bangkok. Leonard Unger was our ambassador there, and the following day a cable came in reply with a quite unorthodox message: "Happy to have Perry and Moune with us." That resolved the question of my next posting.

At the beginning of 1973, I enrolled in the Foreign Service Institute of the State Department for an intensive five-month Thai language training course. There were only a few students in the class, we were all on our way to Bangkok, and we spent hours together five days a week. Once, during recess, I purchased the *Washington Post*, brought it back to the classroom, and noticed that it had a front-page story on Laos with a photo of Prince Souvanna Phouma. A bright young classmate, Janine Brookner, was seated near me at that moment. I pointed to the picture and remarked: "This is my father-in-law." She stared at me with an expression of utter disbelief and then eventually mumbled, "Mm-hmm." I laughed but understood perfectly well her incredulity. I, too, sometimes found it not quite believable.

❊ ❊ ❊

On the morning of February 21, 1973, black official cars began to arrive at the riverside residence of the prime minister, but of the men who emerged from them, only half were members of the government. The others were members of the Pathet Lao.

Prince Souvanna Phouma, ever the genial host, received them inside the house. The large handsome dining room with its crystal chandeliers had been transformed into a meeting room. The men gathered around the long table on which were copies of a pact, one that months of preparation and argument had gone into drafting, and its final version consisted of five chapters and fourteen articles. Pheng Phongsavan, the government's chief negotiator, and Phoumi Vongvichit, a leader of the Pathet Lao, had been designated as the signers of the treaty, and they now proceeded to inscribe their names on the documents. Champagne was served, and Souvanna told the assembled group that peace would permit Laos to progress economically and socially.

The pact was to serve two purposes: to bring a conclusion to the ongoing war, and toward this goal impose an immediate cease-fire throughout the country; and to provide the design for an interim coalition that would lead to a coalition government, the first new coalition government for the kingdom since the one created in Geneva in 1962. The signing of the pact on this February morning was deemed of sufficient importance for *The New York Times* to make the event its three-column lead story on the front page. But while the coalition of 1962 had been a tripartite affair and had divided power among the neutralists, rightists, and communists, this coalition would give the communists a full half partnership. Consequently, as they left the prime minister's residence that morning, the Pathet Lao could hardly contain their smugness if not outright joy. The neutralists seemed for the most part on the defensive, and the rightists appeared disgruntled or bitter.

The pact was complex. It proposed the neutralization of the two government strongholds, Vietiane and Luang Prabang. All soldiers were to leave those two cities and were to be replaced by a police force manned in equal numbers by the government and the Pathet Lao. Cynics claimed it was virtually impossible to distinguish the Pathet Lao police from their soldiers. It was also indicative that there was no suggestion in the pact to neutralize the northern cities held by the Pathet Lao.

Despite the five chapters and fourteen articles, the treaty had failed to be precise about certain substantive matters, and this would lead to additional months of forensic wrangling and negotiation. A paramount question was whether the new coalition was to rule all of the kingdom, including the major part of it, which was under Pathet Lao control, or whether it was to apply solely to that portion which had remained under government control at the beginning of the year.

Yet another prickly issue was one of political innovation. The accord provided for a National Political Coalition Council. The government drafters had intended it to be no more than a supplement to the National Assembly, but there was a suspicious ambiguity about the council that the Pathet Lao had insisted upon.

Why then had Souvanna Shouma accepted such a pact? Under the circumstances, it was the best he could hope for. It was a step toward his desired reunification of the kingdom under his own neutralist leadership. And this step forward was being taken at the very time that the opposition to the communist forces in Southeast Asia was in disarray. The war in South Vietnam was a quagmire. America continued to bombard the Ho Chi Minh Trail in eastern Laos in order to render it unusable as a conduit for supplies from Hanoi to its soldiers in the south, an objective we were never able to realize despite the intensive bombings. But the most formidable threat to the Lao government was the continued presence within the kingdom of some sixty thousand North Vietnamese troops pretending to be Pathet Lao soldiers. Ever since the signing of the 1962 accords, the little kingdom had been under a state of invasion by the North Vietnamese army, and this intolerable situation gave no indication of eventual change.

Before Laos could be completely swallowed up by the North Vietnamese, Souvanna Phouma saw the slim possibility that this new coalition government, despite its inequities, might save, or at least prolong, the life of the kingdom, might even lead to the departure of the Vietnamese forces. He therefore took the risk.

The new agreement would also mean that after many years the Pathet Lao would no longer be the enemy outside the city limits. They would be the enemy within.

◆ ◆ ◆

Five months of Thai language training taught me that what had at first seemed to be a relatively simple tongue proved to be a difficult one in which to achieve fluency. One aspect that deterred my mastery of the language was its tonality. In school when the class would sing, teachers would tell this monotone to be quiet. But the course was eventually completed, and Moune and I impatiently left Washington to return to Asia in the spring of 1973.

En route, we visited with Moune's uncle, who was ambassador to Tokyo. While there, we received a cable from Moune's father. He was eager to see her and asked us to fly from Hong Kong to Vientiane in order to spend the weekend with him before we proceeded to Bangkok. To facilitate these new travel plans, there was a plane of Royal Air Laos, the country's airline, each Saturday from Hong Kong to Vientiane. Approval of this two-day delay in arrival was readily obtained from those concerned in Bangkok.

The Saturday morning on which we were scheduled to leave Hong Kong was dark and stormy. We wondered if the planes were flying. I telephoned the airport and received a vaguely affirmative reply. We took a taxi through the rain to the Hong Kong airport, famous for its landing strips which jut out over the water and for being accessible only by passing between stark, steep hills.

Inside the airport there were few passengers and a somewhat grim ambiance. We checked our luggage at the Royal Air Laos counter, where the pleasant attendant was not very informative. Then we waited. Announcements over the loudspeaking system intermittently pierced the large room. They were of this nature: "Japan Airlines, Flight X, delayed." "Lufthansa, Flight Y canceled." "Pan Am, Flight Z, canceled." And then: "Royal Air Laos, Flight Q to Vientiane, *now boarding*." We looked at each other in dismay. We made our way through the gate to the boarding area and, always hoping it was not going to happen, onto the plane, an old British Viscount. Very few boarded that plane. We were seated in the first row of the first-class section, and a stewardess was most attentive. But we were terribly aware that outside the plane the storm raged on. We fastened our seatbelts with particular care, and the plane roared down the runway and took off. On our way up, the plane shuddered as no plane I have ever been in has done. We clutched each other and believed that our wonderful happiness might be in its last moment. The old Viscount trembled again, a profoundly remorseful movement, and then, incredibly, continued to climb through those menacing, flashing skies until it reached the bright blue above, where a brilliant yellow sun enveloped us in its gloriously welcome light. We sighed. I bent over and kissed my wife and ordered a stiff whiskey.

We arrived in Vientiane on time. Moune's father was waiting for us at his residence, where we spent a fine family reunion weekend and plunged into a discussion of the political situation in the little kingdom.

◆ ◆ ◆

During the year that I had spent in Savannakhet, 1961–1962, I had come to know Colonel Ma, the commander of the Lao air force, which was headquartered at the airport in that city. Often when I went out to the field to meet the incoming milk run flight, I would encounter him and engage in banter with him. He was in his thirties and looked younger. He laughed a lot, joked a lot, and made me somewhat nervous. There was a wildness in his eyes, an implied unpredictability in his behavior. Several times he invited me to fly with him, but the idea of going up in a plane with Ma at the controls did not appeal. I could imagine him going into a series of rolls, loops, and tailspins to entertain—or frighten—me. He was surely not intellectual, but he was political, an ardent supporter of Phoumi Nosavan.

✳ ✳ ✳

When his mentor Phoumi fled to Thailand after a failed coup in 1965, General Thao Ma remained as the head of the air force. He conducted his war against the Pathet Lao with great energy, and his leadership is credited with having hampered the communist advance. But Ma became the subject of rumors and scrutiny, and he was on poor terms with too many of his fellow military officers. It is certain that he strongly resented the general of the army, Kouprasith Abhay, who had broken with Phoumi and eventually pursued Phoumi into exile.

Ma was dismissed as head of the air force in 1966, for what precise reason I do not know. In reaction, in October of that year, he with a small group of followers led an air strike on an army base as part of still another attempted coup. It failed, and now it was Ma's turn to cross the Mekong and remain there in exile.

Phoumi and Ma from their safe haven in Thailand never lost their hopes to reconquer Laos. In their zeal to convert the kingdom into a right-wing dictatorship, they seemed blind to political reality.

In the summer of 1973, while Moune and I were living in a hotel suite in Bangkok as we waited for work to be completed on our house, we learned that Ma had struck again. The negotiations that were underway in Vientiane for the new coalition government so unnerved Ma that he became desperate. Before dawn on the morning of August 20, the general with perhaps five hundred rebel troops crossed into Laos from Thailand. The Mekong was swollen, as it is in that season with a precipitate current, but they got across. Most of them then raced to the Wat Tay airport and secured it, while a small group dashed into town and in predictable fashion captured the radio station. They announced that they were in command, but somehow the people of Vientiane failed to be sufficiently impressed, and the markets and shops remained open for business.

The American ambassador was out of town, and chargé d'affaires John Dean hurried out to the airport to speak to Ma. But the general refused to heed Dean's declaration that the United States would not waive its support for Souvanna Phouma. Ma was not to be dissuaded.

The wildness and unpredictability that I had suspected was within him now surfaced in a highly dramatic and mad action. While his men awaited his orders at Wat Tay airport, Ma climbed into a T–28 plane, took off, flew over the city to Camp Chinaimo, where the army was headquartered, dropped a bomb, and strafed a while, killing several men, then singled out General Kouprasith's house for further strafing, but hit only the kitchen, which was empty at that moment. As Ma, perhaps content with this little sortie, started back to Wat Tay, a government soldier stationed at an anti-aircraft battery spotted, fired upon, and hit his plane. Ma, a brilliant pilot, managed to bring the damaged craft back to the airport but, in his attempt to land, overshot the runway and crashed. And so the irrepressible Ma was fatally repressed.

By then, the government soldiers were advancing on Wat Tay. The rebel forces scattered and were either captured or made their way across the Mekong.

Negotiations for the new coalition government continued.

❋ ❋ ❋

In mid-September 1973, delegates from the Pathet Lao met once more with those from the government at the prime minister's residence in Vientiane as a follow-up to their February meeting. On this occasion they signed the agreement that formally created the new coalition government and expected it to be in operation within a month. In his remarks, Prince Souvanna Phouma declared that there was now an accord among Lao to solve the problems of the kingdom. He said: "We are happy that all Lao are going to have peace and at the same time national reconciliation." He urged his countrymen to maintain a course of international neutrality.

The protocol repeatedly demanded unanimity between the two opposing factions as a prelude to action. It emphasized the role of what was now termed the National Consultative Political Council. Here as an example is Article 9:

> The two parties agree: to confer the responsibility to the National Consultative Political Council, to reexamine and revise and to amend the 1957 law concerning democratic liberties, to adapt them to the current political realities of the country. The National Political Consultative Council must organize democratic general elections in order to consolidate all administrative levels of the state, prepare favorable conditions so that the elections can take place in a truly democratic way to elect a definitive national assembly, achieve national harmony and unify the nation.

When communists riding into power employ such terms as *political realities* and *a truly democratic way*, can we be other than suspicious?

James Markham, who covered the story for *The New York Times*, wrote:

> For the crucial ingredient of goodwill, both sides will have to look to Prince Souvanna Phouma, the durable seventy-two-year-old neutralist.... Paradoxically, Prince Souvanna Phouma's lack of power base will be one of his strengths in the coalition, in which he will be premier once again. Threatening no one, he will be able to appeal to both sides to search for common ground rather than perpetuate fears and suspicion. But the task ahead is enormous.

Those months of intensive language training were not as helpful to me as they might have been. The ministers of education and of culture and the rectors and professors of the universities with whom my work was so largely concerned were all, so it seemed, graduates of Oxford or Cambridge or Berkeley or Harvard, and therefore my weak Thai was no match for their superior English. Nor could I practice Thai with the Fulbright candidates, for they had to prove fluency in English in order to qualify for scholarships. But it was gratifying to be a part of a program which awarded grants not only to sophisticated youngsters of Bangkok but also to bright boys and girls from the rural areas who could not have gone abroad for further education without our assistance.

My limited ability in Thai did allow me to speak with the staff of servants. All of the foreigners in Bangkok had houses with staffs and servants; it was the way of life. That same nineteenth-century style extended to tennis at the Royal Bangkok Sports Club, where there were grass courts, obligatory white dress, and ball boys to retrieve any errant white tennis balls.

Ours was a large old-fashioned house with a lawn that stretched what appeared to be the length of a football field down to a busy canal, on which boats noisily scuttled along day and night. Occasionally our cook would hail a boat to take her to market; other times, merchants would tie up at our dock to sell the magnificent fruits and vegetables they were transporting on the water. The long green lawn adapted itself readily to parties and once to a classical concert offered by the resident American string quartet. On one side were trees with wild orchids growing from their trunks and branches, on the other side a large cluster of poinsettias, some of them over fifteen feet high and all of them a brilliant red for Christmas. On top of the garage was a very large bedroom and bath. We initially paid scant attention to what seemed an unnecessary additional apartment, but during our four years there it proved to be of tremendous value to us for reasons that will become evident.

Bangkok may have been insufferably hot and its traffic horrendous, but living in that city was utterly delightful. Those Thais with whom we formed lasting friendships were intelligent, charming, and witty. Since Moune was of a family looked upon as cousins of sort, we were often entertained by members of the royal family. One, Princess Chumbhot of Nagor Svarga, was brilliant and extraordinary; strong-willed with a wicked sense of humor, she was a joy to be with. While we were there, she founded the first museum for modern art in Thailand, a handsome structure designed by her Harvard-trained architect nephew, and Moune and I were among the original members of its board.

Once each month we spent a weekend in Vientiane. Moune's brother Panya was the director of Royal Air Lao, and that facilitated our arrangements for transportation there and back. We would stay with my father-in-law, and on those weekends when we were not involved in social activities we would spend simple, memorable evenings of dinner and bridge at home. Prince Souvanna Phouma rarely allowed himself to reveal how troubled he was by the problems of the new coalition government.

During this period he took great pleasure in employing his architectural training to design and build a new house in Luang Prabang, where he planned eventually to retire. It was a solid, spacious house where the comfort of the inhabitants and visitors was being meticulously prepared for. Five large bedrooms and baths were on the second floor.

When the house was completed, the blessings of the monks became a major event, and Their Majesties came to assist. The furniture was removed from the large salon, and the floor was covered by rugs, on which we all sat with our legs to one side while the *bonzes* intoned their prayers. Because this was a special house and the king and queen were present, the monks went on at great length—for almost three hours. My recollection of that morning is rather acute since unlike the dear Lao with whom I sat and by whom I was surrounded, I could not position my legs in a way that after a while would be other than painful. I tried as unobtrusively as I could to move them in one way or another, to find a direction in which I might straighten them out without kicking some of the good people about me. I even tried kneeling inconspicuously, but nothing helped. And one simply could not get up and leave the room while Their Majesties were there. At last the monks completed their blessings. I was in a sorry state and with difficulty struggled up on my unsteady feet.

A gala open house that evening also went on for many hours, during which I was not confined to the floor and was able to maneuver from one room to the next, from one glass to another, with much enjoyment.

◆ ◆ ◆

A certain current practice in Southeast Asia if it is mentioned here in the West is apt to be misunderstood. There, when a man and woman are without offspring and one of the couple has a sister or brother with several or numerous children, one of these nephews or nieces will be given to the childless couple. A strong sense of family prevails in that part of the world, and the transfer of a child from one sibling to another is not considered a sacrifice but simply an altogether logical implementation of the family. The adopted child is not cut off from his parents but fully accepts his legal parents as his very own. The result is that while some are enriched, no one feels deprived.

Moune's brother, Prince Mangkhara, and his wife Princess Ouanna, a niece of the king, had four children, of whom the eldest, Daraphon, was a most vivacious little girl who spent much time in Vientiane living with her grandfather, the prime minister. Prince Souvanna often spoke of Dara as a young Moune. She did resemble her Aunt Moune, and when Moune returned from Paris to be at the Ministry of Foreign Affairs, the two spent much time together. After Moune and I were married and moved into the ranch house, the first visitor to occupy the guest room was Dara.

Years later when we were in Bangkok, Dara came to spend her school vacation. And Prince Souvanna declared that the girl should be a member of the Stieglitz family. Mangkhara and Ouanna agreed, and Dara was asked if the proposal appealed to her. Feeling as close as she did to Moune, she readily accepted to become our daughter. At that time, she was ten years old.

We formally adopted her, and she was a lively, sometimes boisterous addition to our Bangkok household. Coquelicot, our superintelligent white miniature poodle, accepted her as a sister, and the good Thai servants made a fine fuss in welcoming her. We sent her to the French school so that she could continue her studies in that language.

Moune and I were happy that this lovely tradition existed.

❀ ❀ ❀

The new coalition government that was to have been functional by October of 1973 actually came into existence on the second day of April in 1974. The event was shrewdly planned by Prince Souphanouvong. On that day he made his first return to Vientiane in a decade, and his arrival was staged as a major celebration. Two thousand persons were at Wat Tay airport when he flew in from the north. As he descended from the plane, the crowd cheered the "Red Prince." His half-brother, Prince Souvanna Phouma, was waiting on the tarmac, and the two warmly embraced. Members of the diplomatic corps, including the American ambassador, were also on the scene. After greetings and fanfare, Souphanouvong left for the city in a convoy of Pathet Lao soldiers.

A cabinet was soon announced with Souvanna as prime minister and two deputy prime ministers, one from Vientiane and the other of the Pathet Lao. Sisouk na Champassak and Ngon Sananikone remained as members of the cabinet, the former as the new minister of defense, Ngon as minister of finance. The Pathet Lao had insisted that one of their own be the new minister of foreign affairs, a choice that gravely troubled concerned Westerners. But the major surprise was that Souphanouvong rejected the role of deputy prime minister and chose instead to head the new National Consultative Political Council, which was to consist of sixteen members of the Pathet Lao, sixteen from the combined neutralist-rightist faction, and ten to be approved by both sides.

Once more Vientiane became a center of international intrigue, and the bar of the Hotel Constellation was again crowded. In the region where the war against the communists was so desperate, the little kingdom was proclaiming itself to be a neutralist nation with communist and anticommunists participating on what were supposedly equal terms. Worldwide attention was focused here, and the overriding question was: Could a coalition with the communists succeed?

Moune and I spent a weekend in June with her father at the house in Luang Prabang, where one evening Souphanouvong joined us for dinner. He was as affable as ever, although undeniably more pretentious. In the past, he had often enjoyed his bridge game and played it skillfully, but now he felt it incumbent upon himself to renounce this bourgeois pastime. Therefore, after dinner, instead of playing cards, we sat about on the large rear veranda, my father-in-law puffing on a large cigar, some of us sipping whiskey, and Uncle Souphanouvong doing most of the talking. He described with enthusiasm the cultural activities of the Lao in Pathet Lao territories and how they formed dance groups and improvised entertainments. But what I remember most distinctly, and have had reason to remember regretfully ever since, was his positive statement that the Pathet Lao people held Their Majesties in great reverence and would never harm them.

That evening Souphanouvong could well afford to be cocky. The two months since he had returned to Vientiane had been good ones for him. He had been busy molding the National Political Council into the seat of power for the government. He did not object that a key provision of the new constitution that all foreign troops were to leave was being blatantly ignored by the North Vietnamese soldiers, estimated to be more than fifty thousand in number. Sisouk, the minister of defense, declared that these soldiers had "withdrawn into the scenery but not back home."

In May, the new cabinet, mandated to function on the principle of unanimity, had denied permission for the National Assembly to hold its traditional opening ceremonies. True, the National Assembly, a holdover from the previous government, consisted exclusively of rightists and neutralists, but only because through the years the Pathet Lao had refused to elect representatives. Most members of the Assembly, in reaction to this lethal blow struck against it, expressed outrage, but a few joined the leftist power machine. Souphanouvong hinted at the eventual establishment of a new and "legal" National Assembly.

The Pathet Lao soldiers were very much in evidence in Luang Prabang. Perhaps this offered Prince Souphanouvong a sense of security, and this may be why he chose the beautiful royal capital, in preference to Vientiane, as the base for his National Political Council.

The neutralist policies Prince Souvanna Phouma had nurtured so astutely for so many years were under the fiercest of attacks.

◆ ◆ ◆

Political tensions mounted in Vientiane. Two members of the National Assembly attempted to distribute a petition of protest against the continued presence of North Vietnamese soldiers on Lao soil, and the two were promptly arrested by Pathet Lao soldiers. An embattled cabinet met in a heated, sometimes unruly session on Tuesday, July 10, 1974, and remained assembled until the prime minister was able to obtain a unanimous decision to dissolve the National Assembly. That the assembly was a holdover from the previous anticommunist regime made it an anachronism. Nevertheless, it was a difficult and unwelcome task that Prince Souvanna Phouma had had to undertake, and it put him under abnormal stress.

Two days later, about to leave on a visit to the University of Hat Yai in southern Thailand, I persuaded Moune to join me with the promise that we could spend the weekend at the nearby town of Songkhla on the Gulf of Siam. That is where we were on Friday evening when we received an urgent call to return to Bangkok; Moune's father, we were told, was gravely ill after having suffered cardiac arrest.

At the airport early the next morning, we learned that the two flights scheduled for Bangkok that day were completely booked. We waited, hoped, and prayed and got on the first flight. Two Americans from our embassy were waiting for us at the Bangkok airport, and they rushed Moune on to a special plane for Vientiane.

I took care of matters that demanded attention at our house and at my office and several days later joined Moune in Vientiane.

She met me at Wat Tay and we drove to her father's residence. The parking space was crowded, and we had to make our way through soldiers, journalists, and officials. Inside the family house was the quiet, the soft voices, and the smell of medicines that one associated with illness. I was relieved to note that the military officer was there to prevent any unauthorized person from going up the stairs.

We left my baggage in our room, and I was admitted to my father-in-law's room. The blinds were drawn, and only the light from one small lamp pierced the dimness. The prince was stretched out on a hospital bed. He was pale and obviously weak. I stepped to his side, he looked up at me, and he nodded. With feeble motions, he signaled the nurse to him and conveyed a message to her. She brought a chair from the other side of the room and placed it next to his bed, then told me His Highness wished me to sit there. I did so. The prince stretched out his hand to me, and I clasped it for a moment. Then we spent I do not know how much time—he drowsy, occasionally napping—I silently by his side. Here was my second father in this frighteningly delicate condition.

My brother-in-law, Prince Mangkhara, suggested that I join the conference to be held in the official dining room of the residence late that afternoon. This, I learned, was a daily ritual. Seated around the long table were some twenty persons, all of whom expect for members of the family were doctors or interpreters. In addition to the two Lao doctors there were a leading heart specialist from Bangkok, whom the Thai government had rushed to the scene, and a young, brilliant American cardiologist from Clark Field in the Philippines, who represented a contribution from the

United States government. The French doctor in residence in Laos had been joined by two heart men flown in from Paris. The Soviet Union sent three specialists to tend to the prime minister, and three Chinese physicians—an elderly gentleman and two intense women—came from Beijing as an offering from the People's Republic of China. Surely this was a unique event in the annals of international medicine.

At the end of each afternoon, these doctors gathered about the dining room table would discuss and argue what the latest examinations of the patient had revealed, what remedies should be applied, what should be avoided. I was anything but amused at the thought of United Nations delegates trying to resolve unanimously a current and urgent crisis.

Even during the days I was there, the dining room sessions were growing progressively longer, for each country had to make medical points, and additional interpreters were required. The doctors were lodged at their respective embassies or at the Lan Xang Hotel, but all of them each evening immediately following the "committee" meeting took dinner with the family at the prime minister's residence. This gave us the occasion to become acquainted with them. I noticed that among themselves they engaged for the most part in polite and sometimes amiable conversations, with one notable exception: the Russians and the Chinese deliberately avoided each other.

Despite the ministrations of this often contentious group, the prince made satisfactory progress. I returned to Bangkok some days later, but Moune remained in Vientiane.

News of Souvanna Phouma's heart attack reverberated throughout that part of the world concerned with the affairs of Southeast Asia. A *New York Times* editorial on July 23 was headlined "Indispensable Laotian" and explained: "Prince Souvanna Phouma is the indispensable man who alone is believed able both to hold the coalition government together—and to make it work. . . . But, unless the Premier makes a rapid recovery, Laos will soon be headed into the unknown." That five countries which supported opposing factions in the war in the region had sent eminent doctors to do whatever was possible to aid Souvanna indicated the importance they placed on the survival of this man. And this was another remarkable instance of virtual unanimity among the world's great powers on the subject of a tiny, weak kingdom.

The cardiac arrest also brought to a temporary hold the growing friction between the former Lao government leaders and their new partner, the Pathet Lao. On July 27, Prince Souphanouvong and other leftist officials met for the first time with those rightists who had long been their enemies to seek some reconciliation in the light of the prime minister's illness. The meeting succeeded to a surprising measure.

There was friction as might have been expected as to the choice of which of the two deputy prime ministers would be acting premier during Souvanna's incapacitation. Here Souphanouvong, who spent much time with his stricken half-brother, prevailed, and the Pathet Lao, Phoumi Vongvichit, was announced as Souvanna's choice. This decision was made in August before the patient left for what was to have been a month's recovery abroad. In the selection of a country to which he should go, Souphanouvong was again influential, for the United States invited Souvanna to go there for his convalescence, but the Pathet Lao preferred that he go to France, and so to France he went.

He traveled aboard a French military hospital plane, and Moune accompanied him. The plane developed engine trouble over Egypt, made an emergency landing, and the prince and Moune were transferred to another French army plane to complete the voyage. But Moune's baggage had been left behind in Egypt. I groaned a bit but was also somewhat amused at the idea of my darling fashion-conscious wife arriving in France with literally nothing to wear other than what she had on.

Moune stayed with her father for a month, by which time he had made a good recovery. She then came back to Bangkok.

To the surprise of many and the relief of most, the coalition government remained intact and functioning. The little kingdom was indicating that perhaps it could survive as a more or less neutralist nation into an indefinite future.

The prince returned from France in October and was given a tumultuous welcome by Prince Souphanouvong and the thousands who waited for his plane at Wat Tay airport. The cardiac *cause célèbre* affirmed the admiration and abiding affection of his people for Souvanna Phouma and was to a large measure responsible for this interval of good will.

Moune and I had our own private reunion with the great man. But we knew he was not yet fully recovered. He wanted to wait a while longer before returning to the bridge table.

❊ ❊ ❊

The brave front and crowded social scene that had been such an integral part of life in Vientiane continued into the early months of 1975. However, the rapidly deteriorating conditions in South Vietnam and Cambodia placed untenable pressures on the delicate coalition government. For years a principal supporter of Prince Souvanna Phouma's attempts to sustain a neutralist administration, the United States was now reducing its financial aid and even its interest. America's fiercely criticized involvement in South Vietnam had left no room for concern about little Laos. The prince seemed to be his confident and reassuring self, but those of us who knew him well realized how deeply distressed he was and feared for his recently recovered health.

The military activities of the combined Pathet Lao–North Vietnamese armies had been for a while relatively quiet, but by April those soldiers resumed their expansionist march within the kingdom. Near the end of the month, they chose to attack the government-held village and airport of Sala Phou Khoun, almost one hundred miles north of Vientiane. Consequently, this became the site for the little kingdom's last military stand. Sisouk na Champassak was a most determined minister of defense. He was definitely in charge of his armies. When the enemy forced the government soldiers to retreat from Sala Phou Khoun under a barrage of artillery attacks on April 23, Sisouk had his troops regroup and recapture the village on April 28, the same day that the American embassy was being evacuated in Saigon.

Sisouk surely knew how slight was the possibility of eventual success against the North Vietnamese, yet he felt compelled to continue the armed battle. Souvanna, ever faithful to his own convictions, was determined not to have his country engage in another bloody civil war, one in which his army was no match for the North Vietnamese juggernaut. Souvanna and Sisouk argued at length, Sisouk more emotional, Souvanna more reasonable, and each had sympathy for the other's objections. Souvanna prevailed, and Sisouk resigned from the cabinet. The prince, always with compassion for his people, hoped to resolve the conflict by compromise. He himself was, after all, the acknowledged master of solving national crises through political means, and he counted on his half brother and the Pathet Lao to maintain their allegiance to the king.

The great exodus from the kingdom started at the end of April. Among the first to flee were the thousands of Chinese and Vietnamese who had made their home in Laos. Thousands of Lao who had opposed the communist takeover correctly surmised that they were targeted for prison camps or worse and made their way across the river to Thailand. The American families were evacuated, then most of the American officials.

With the fall of Saigon, the North Vietnamese were in full command of what had been Indochina. They did not, however, immediately proclaim themselves masters of Laos. They preferred to play a game of sorts that lasted for months and during which they gradually announced the changes they had already made.

Rather than directly dissolve the government that had been established by the Geneva accords, the Pathet Lao employed various stratagems. One of these was inciting students in vast numbers to stage protests against the rightists and the Americans, but anyone who knew the Lao students was aware that these manifestations were artificial and completely alien to the gentle nature of Lao youth.

By early June, all the Americans except for twenty-two attached to the embassy had left the country. Many of the Pathet Lao wished to close down the embassy, but Souvanna Phouma, no longer prime minister but named advisor to the new government, won his argument that the American presence must be permitted. The American embassy, headed by a chargé d'affaires, remains in Vientiane even as this is written.

Prince Souvanna Phouma played an extraordinary role during the transition of Laos from a kingdom to a communist vassal-state. The fight he had fought for many years to keep his small country independent and neutralist, and out of communist control, had been lost. He had an apartment in Paris and a home in southern France to which he could have retired. He had had his previous year's heart attack as a valid reason for him to remove himself from the scene. But Souvanna Phouma refused to take the easy exit afforded to him. He had been the leader of his people through extreme difficulties, and he refused to abandon them now. It is in large measure thanks to his remaining on the scene that the death of the little kingdom was not accompanied by any grim scenes of slaughter and bloodshed.

◆ ◆ ◆

Not that Souvanna Phouma was able to prevent the new government from systematically wreaking its vengeance against those who had legitimately opposed their coming to power and who had the misfortune to remain in Laos. So-called reeducation camps were established in the north, and those who had been the leaders of the rightist movements, the generals, the intellectuals, were told they were being sent to these camps for a period of indoctrination. Most of those who were sent to these camps—labor camps where they were forced to work in the fields throughout daylight hours, were miserably housed and fed little more than starvation diets—died there, some of them, according to reports, beaten to death. My good friend, General Boun Pone of Savannakhet was among these. Moune's dear friend, Khamchan Pradit, was serving as ambassador to Australia when he was summoned home by the new communist government. He spoke to Moune, she urged him not to go back to Vientiane, but he felt it was his duty to do so and that furthermore, as a good civil servant, he had nothing to fear from the government. He returned to Vientiane and was promptly sent up to a reeducation camp from which he has not returned.

* * *

By the end of 1975, all pretense was gone, and the Pathet Lao ruled with my uncle, Prince Souphanouvong, as president of the People's Republic of Laos.

Souphanouvong had vowed that no harm would befall Their Majesties under the Pathet Lao. Within the year, the king, the queen, and the crown prince were all sent up north. An entirely reliable witness tells us that the king was sent to a camp, where he was treated as brutally as were the other prisoners. No special treatment was accorded him. According to this witness, who was also a prisoner at that camp, the king and the crown prince died within several days of each other.

◆ ◆ ◆

And in this way, the lovely little kingdom reached its ignoble ending.

◆ ◆ ◆

Imagine that you live in the country of your ancestors, that the political party to which you belong loses an election, and that, as a result, you have to flee from your home and country to save your life, taking with you few or no possessions. In Laos, of course, it was more than political parties, it was ideologies; and it was more than an election, it was a military takeover preceded by elections. Nevertheless, the analogy suggests itself, and is chilling.

Our spare apartment in Bangkok had been largely vacant for two years but suddenly seemed essential.

First it was a cousin, a young woman with three children who managed to get to Thailand. Her husband had been killed in the fighting, and she had to wait until the necessary papers came through before she could continue to France. She occupied the apartment for several weeks.

Then other cousins.

The French wife of a son of Prince Khammao and Princess Khamla arrived from France. She anxiously waited with us for her husband to get out of Laos. Eventually he did.

Other members of the family came, some for brief periods. Those without funds faced internment in the refugee camps, and we naturally tried to help them avoid that.

Prince Panya, Moune's brother, had chosen to stay with his father in Vientiane. In November of 1975, he learned that on the following day he was going to be sent north to a reeducation camp. That night, Panya placed his passport and other vital papers in waterproof wrapping put them in a money belt, and tied the belt around him. He dressed himself for immersion and covered his body with grease. The Mekong at that time was almost at flood level, and its powerful current carried swiftly downstream all manners of debris. Fortunately, Panya was an outstanding athlete and still in his prime. Near midnight, he slipped into the treacherous river and spent the next several hours struggling through the racing waters. As he swam, he could not be certain of his direction, for the currents, the litter, and the floating lumber had him spinning. When at last, weak but determined, he reached land and climbed up the shore, he did not know whether he had crossed the river or had been swept back to Laos. Soon he was spotted and led to the nearby border police headquarters, where he was at once recognized.

Moune and I had invited a dozen friends for Thanksgiving dinner. We particularly wanted our daughter, Dara, to participate in this most American of holidays. Early that morning, I received a telephone call from the editor-in-chief of the *Bangkok Post*, who informed me in breathless tones of Panya's accomplishment. Late that afternoon, Panya reached Bangkok and came directly to our house, where his wife, who had been waiting for him in this city, joined us and our friends in a Thanksgiving Day celebration for which we were more than thankful.

Within months, Moune's other brother, Prince Mangkhara and his wife, Princess Ouanna, and their three children realized that they were courting danger if they remained in their own country. But they were a family unit and had to move as one. To make their escape, they were able to hire—or bribe—a Thai boatman to transport them across the Mekong on another dark night.

For the next month or more, Mangkhara and his family occupied the apartment, Panya and his wife one of our bedrooms. The house was crowded, but there were no complaints.

Moune and I were grateful for my having been posted to Bangkok and our being able to render some small service to these courageous refugees.

◆ ◆ ◆

Before my four-year assignment to Bangkok came to an end in 1977, a cable announced that my next post was to be cultural attaché in Brussels. Excellent cable! Having programmed the Alvin Ailey Dance Company for Thailand that summer and having to be on hand for their performances and the many surrounding activities, I encouraged Moune and Dara not to wait for me, for they wanted to visit the family in France, to select a school for Dara, and to find housing for us in Belgium.

Soon after they had gone, I walked down the street from my office to the nearby Lao embassy. Until the events of 1975, I had known the Lao ambassador and several of his aides. Now I entered an uninviting chancery where I knew no one and where visas were begrudgingly granted, and rarely to Americans. As I filled out the application form, I smiled at its final question: What is your reason for going to the People's Republic of Laos? I wrote: To visit members of my family.

The young official who took my application read it and made no comment. I decided that the prime purpose for the chancery was to allow its bureaucrats to indulge in delaying tactics. But the fourth time I returned to ask for my visa, it was granted to me. Obviously, someone with influence in Laos had intervened on my behalf.

As I prepared for my weekend in Vientiane, I received a telephone call from the Netherlands ambassador to Bangkok: he wanted to see me. He was also accredited as the envoy to Laos—it is a common practice for a major embassy to cover small neighboring countries. In his office he told me that he had just come back from Vientiane and had some disturbing news to report to me: my father-in-law, he said, had changed and had become a communist sympathizer. I lacked the evidence to refute—or agree with—this comment.

No commercial planes flew in the period between Bangkok and Vientiane, but the overnight trains to the Thai village nearest Vientiane had a certain wayward charm. The American chargé d'affaires to Laos, the amiable Tom Corcoran was notified by our embassy in Bangkok that I was arriving for the weekend. That is why on that Friday morning, after I got off the train, checked through Thai customs, descended the steep Mekong embankment, boarded a *pirogue* that bumped its way across the river, climbed up the Lao side, and checked through Lao customs, I was greeted by one of the American officers at our embassy there who was making certain that I would encounter no unforeseen difficulties between the customs shed and my father-in-law's residence.

The prince was waiting for me and greeted me warmly. Visitors to Vientiane at that time were such a rare occurrence that my presence became something of an event. He had a servant take my bag up to the bedroom that had been prepared for me. His sister, Princess Khamla, one of my favorite aunts, was living at the residence, and she and I had a most cordial reunion.

We had lunch in the dining room with two other cousins. The ladies had strong reasons to be unhappy with the privations they were enduring, but no one complained. On the contrary, it was a jolly occasion, and conversation was lively and often witty.

After lunch we were suddenly confronted by ominous reality. My father-in-law's faithful aide came into the salon as we were drinking coffee and, excusing himself profusely, explained that it was necessary for him to speak with the prince. They spoke in Lao, and I was unable to follow much of the discussion, but I saw my father-in-law grow vexed. After a while he turned to me and told me it had been requested (who had made the request was never specified) that I not stay at the residence but should instead be lodging with one of the Americans. The residence of the American chargé, previously the American ambassador's, was not far, and Tom had already kindly asked if I wished to stay with him; therefore, the demand presented no problem for me. The prince, however, felt a humiliation of sorts that he was not allowed to have his son-in-law remain at his home with him. I tried to make light of the matter and did not refer to it again, but this was the only instance I can remember when his pride had been visibly hurt.

One of my father-in-law's cars and his chauffeur were placed at my disposal to facilitate going back and forth between the two residences. On Saturday morning, not wishing to telephone for the driver and enjoying the idea of stretching my legs, I walked from the American residence to the family home. My father-in-law's aide, a fine, gentle Lao with no trace of arrogance, saw me arrive. He was nervous. He told me softly but firmly that I must not walk between the two houses and made me assure him that I would not repeat that little promenade. To render the ban less severe, he promised to take me for a ride that afternoon into town and along the river, for he knew I was deeply curious about what changes might be taking place.

That summer, Vientiane was the most moribund city I have ever seen and certainly ever hope to see. As we drove through the streets where the shops had flourished, we were greeted by an emptiness and silence that were chilling. No people were at the afternoon market. I caught only one glimpse of monks—there were four of them. We drove along the river beyond the boundaries of the city and saw one factory and one lumber mill where work was going on, but I saw virtually no other activity. I remarked on the large loudspeakers hoisted onto the poles carrying the wires for electricity. These speakers, I was told, were used to get the people out of their houses early in the mornings and onto the streets for physical exercise drills. How those quiet sensitive people must have suffered through such treatment.

Friday evening, most of Saturday, and Sunday morning, the prince and I were alone and engaged in a lengthy verbal recapitulation of the history of the little kingdom. Absolutely contrary to what the Dutch ambassador had told me, Souvanna Phouma's keen mind remained brilliantly clear and extraordinarily objective.

When he was prime minister in 1960, Americans had armed and aided his enemy, Phoumi Nosavan, the vicious hard-line rightist who overthrew the prince's legitimate government in the bloody Battle of Vientiane. Then the American administration changed, and when for more than a year the fourteen nations met and negotiated in Geneva on the subject of Laos, the Americans, under his friend, Averell Harriman, had been his most stalwart supporters. The prince was fully aware that during the Vietnamese war some of the American military leadership were discontent with his neutrality, even to the point of planning action against him. But again he fully appreciated the great assistance offered to him by the United States government. Finally, after he recovered from his heart attack and the situation rapidly worsened in South Vietnam, he had watched the Americans' interest in him and support for his cause diminish. All of this he was entirely aware of and, remarkably, understood. He was neither a bitter critic nor an all-out defender of the United States. He and his political cause had been both buffeted and aided by our country.

Similarly, he took keen cognizance of the relations his government had had with the other powers. Some commentators on the international scene claim that Souvanna Phouma was one of the most astute political figures of his time. Without denying this, I found that as a man he was above politics. His was more of a philosophical intellect, and he was forever a devout Buddhist.

It was surely nonsense to believe, as did the Dutch ambassador, that the prince had been persuaded by his brother and the communist regime in Laos to become one of them. No such thing. On the contrary, he was completely aware of how the Pathet Lao had been persistently deceitful: how they had violated every arrangement and treaty they had entered into; how they had plotted the overthrow of the elected government; how they had been willingly exploited by the North Vietnamese. Souvanna Phouma had not for an instant forgotten. By his choosing to continue to live in communist Laos, many assumed that he had forgotten or forgiven the past.

His friendly, positive view of the United States was decidedly influenced by his friendship with Harriman. It also helped that an American had become a very close member of his immediate family.

On Sunday, as I was preparing to leave Vientiane, Princess Khamla called me into her room to ask a favor. She saw little or no possibility of her ever leaving Laos and had some precious rings, necklaces, and bracelets that she wanted her children in France to have. She had wrapped these carefully together in a silk envelope. Could I, she asked, take them with me and bring them to Paris? The many possible dangers in such an act leaped into mind: I was going to be smuggling jewelry, and as a diplomat, if caught, my career would come to a prompt and ignominious conclusion. And yet the action I was being asked to perform was not wrong but was entirely justifiable. Furthermore, I could not say no to this splendid woman, whom I admired so much.

An hour later I said goodbye to my father-in-law and to Princess Khamla with the family jewels concealed in the undershorts in my bag.

Two months later the jewelry was safely delivered to her children in Paris.

◆ ◆ ◆

We worried about the condition of Souvanna Phouma and what degree of freedom he enjoyed in the authoritarian state that Laos had become. Therefore, we felt some relief when in the years after my weekend with him he traveled twice to France. On each occasion he took care of personal matters, including health and finances, and spent time with the family, including Moune, who joined him there. He accepted an invitation to lunch at the Palais des Champs Elysées with President Giscard-d'Estaing. He certainly had the opportunity to declare that he wished to stay in France, where he had an apartment in Paris and a house on the Côte d'Azur, but such an action never seemed to have occurred to him. He never tarried long in France and each time returned directly to Laos. He was not, however, completely free during these overseas visits, for the Vientiane government had one of its "aides" accompany him. The "aide" was a silent observer even during the family gatherings, casting a pall.

Moune and Dara went back to Laos during the school vacation of 1982. This was a happy reunion for father, daughter, and granddaughter. Vientiane by then was in a less depressed condition than it had been five years earlier, and Moune was able to meet with some family and friends who where still there—and alive. The prince had always had a special fondness for Dara and was enthralled to see how his little girl had grown into an attractive young lady. My wife and daughter complained that under these circumstances the two weeks passed with unbecoming rapidity.

We were living in Washington in October of 1984 when Moune received a telephone call from her brother Panya in Bangkok. He told her that their father, according to reports, was gravely ill. Within twenty-four hours Moune had packed her bags and left for Bangkok, where she stayed with our dear friends Tim and Fran Lewis. However, her numerous and repeated demands to enter Laos were denied.

Moune is persistent and not easily defeated. By early December she telephoned me and declared that while she was continuing her efforts to get to see her father, Dara and I were to come to Bangkok to join her for the holidays. That winter was something of a low point for me financially. I was not working and was just making ends meet, so the idea of adding to our expenses by this unexpected voyage halfway around the earth was somewhat disconcerting. The situation was made easier by dear Tim and

Fran insisting the three of us were to be their house guests during the holiday period. Accordingly, the day the school semester ended, Dara and I flew off to Asia.

The three of us presented ourselves at the Lao chancery with new demands for visas. By then, those in the visa section knew well who we were. A week went by, then a second, and we were meeting only with the same delaying tactics.

It was necessary for Dara to return to school in January, and we had our firm reservations for the return flight. Moune planned to go back with us, and the time to leave was approaching. Then the chancery informed us that Dara, and Dara alone, was granted a visa. Frantic visits to the Lao embassy in Bangkok and phone calls gotten through with much difficulty to the Ministry of Foreign Affairs in Vientiane conveyed the message that we would not allow Dara to travel to Laos unless I accompanied her. Our protests resulted in my also being granted a visa. The time left would allow us to spend four days in Vientiane if we returned to Bangkok on the same day that we were scheduled to depart for home, and that is what we arranged to do.

The morning that Moune took us to the airport to take the plane to Laos, I felt extraordinarily sad for her. We tried to imagine why the Lao government so adamantly refused to allow her to visit her ill father, and assumed that her uncle Souphanouvong, then president of the People's Republic of Laos, did not want her there. Later our suspicions were more or less confirmed when we learned that Souphanouvong had made himself executor of his half-brother's estate and that the considerable sums of money that had been willed to each of Souvanna Phouma's grandchildren had been appropriated by the president and no doubt had gone into his personal Swiss bank account. He certainly did not want Moune on the scene to ask questions about her father's will.

The American ambassador to Bangkok, John Gunther Dean, had himself served in Laos and was concerned and helpful to our plight. He sent word to the American chargé in Vientiane, who kindly invited me to stay again at her residence, an invitation I at once accepted because of my previous experience and because I did not want to impose on Princess Khamla, who remained at my father-in-law's tending to his needs. Dara, though, slept in her grandfather's home.

When we arrived at the Wat Tay airport, my father-in-law's driver and another young man were waiting for us and drove us to the house, where Princess Khamla greeted us. She led us upstairs and into the prince's room. After he had suffered his heart attack, I had been distressed to see him but hopeful for his recovery. That was very different from this time, for when I looked at his once solid body reduced to little more than a skeletal frame, hope vanished. He was dying. However, he was alert and happy to see Dara and me. Despite his fragile condition, that afternoon I was able to converse with him for a short while. I told him that Moune was in Bangkok—did he know—and that it would still be possible for her to join us if she could obtain a visa. I thought he listened sympathetically. I left the room and Dara, who had been a volunteer nurse's aide for two summers, used her experience to fuss about her grandfather and to massage his arms and legs.

The Soviet doctor attending the prince called to see his patient and spoke with me afterward. He told me that the prince's heart was faring poorly and that the prince could not survive more than another two to three months. Nevertheless, having known others who have succumbed to cancer that so wholly diminished their bodies and ate away their flesh, I believed that my father-in-law was suffering from some such manner of disease rather than from a heart condition, which more often tends to kill with blessed speed.

At the chargé's home that evening, my thoughts kept returning to my bedside conversation and made me confident that the next day I would be able to persuade my father-in-law to send for Moune despite any objections from others, meaning particularly Souphanouvong.

The next morning, though, when I returned to his house and entered his room, my heart sank, for the prince appeared to be far weaker than he had been on the previous day. I wondered, had he roused himself from his failing state to greet his granddaughter? Or had her visit energized him briefly? The others in attendance, including Princess Khamla and the doctor, did not remark any difference in his condition, but I definitely did. Sadly, most sadly, the conversation I was planning to have on the subject of getting Moune to Vientiane simply could not take place. His condition would not permit.

The president of the republic was out of town, but his very North Vietnamese wife, Viengkham, who kept careful note of what was happening in Souvanna's home, learned that I was there and announced she was coming by to see me.

One of her sons—they had numerous children—had been living at his Uncle Souvanna's, preferring to be there with his Aunt Khamla rather than at his parents' house. He was a bright young man who wanted to distance himself from his mother. When he learned she was coming, he disappeared into his room and locked himself in until after she had gone.

Viengkham arrived, an attractive, vigorous woman, absolutely sure of herself. She greeted me amicably; we had met on several previous occasions, and, as Moune's husband, I was an object of particular interest. We sat in the family living room and had tea. She asked many questions with political implications about America. I had no reluctance to advance pro-American viewpoints with which she was certain to disagree. One bit of conversation is indelible in my memory. We were speaking French, and she, not pleased with my arguments, stated: "At last, the Lao people have been liberated." To which I immediately replied: "*Au contraire.*" That was a sassy reply which gave me an instant satisfaction, but it was made without forethought and could have had unpleasant repercussions for me. She did pause, as though deciding how to react—did she ask herself, should I have this American scoundrel thrown in jail?—then let it pass and continued in her praise for all things communist.

When she left, Princess Khamla said to me, "she's a dangerous woman." Viengkham's son, coming out of hiding, did not say as much but surely was of the same opinion.

The third day the prince was weaker still, and no conversation could take place.

On the fourth morning, Dara and I went into his room to say goodbye. He was a little more alert and wished us a good trip home.

We were delivered to Wat Tay airport by the same driver and his companion who had been with me every time I stepped foot out of the American or my father-in-law's residence. After we had checked through passport control, Dara asked: "How did you like your bodyguard, Daddy?"

I looked at her, clearly puzzled by the question.

She laughed, and then continued as though to an unsuspecting child: "Daddy, surely you knew that the young man who was with the driver was your bodyguard?"

I felt stupidly naive. I had never questioned why that young fellow was always there.

Moune joined us at the Bangkok airport, and the three of us flew on to Tokyo, or more precisely Narita, where we had to spend the night at an airport hotel before embarking on our nonstop Tokyo–New York flight the next day. We had dinner at the hotel and afterwards took a walk about in the vicinity. As we returned to the lobby, one of the hotel clerks came from behind the desk to tell us we had received an urgent phone call and were to telephone Tim Lewis in Bangkok. We did so, and Tim informed us that Moune's father had died a few hours after Dara and I had left him.

We wept and wondered whether or not to return to Bangkok. But Buddhist funerals, especially for prominent men, may take place many weeks after the death. Furthermore, and the deciding factor, there was no certainty that any of us would receive a visa to return to Laos. The next day, as scheduled, the three of us boarded the plane which would take us back to America.

The little kingdom had ceased to be in 1975. Prince Souvanna Phouma stayed on for nine years after all that he had hoped to achieve for his kingdom had failed. He had made easier the transition for his people from the government he had led to the one he had adamantly opposed. The prince was a great patriot who loved his gentle people and remained united with them until death.

Index

PERRY STIEGLITZ presently represents Gibraltar in Washington, D.C. He did his graduate studies at the University of Lausanne, Switzerland. In 1959, Mr. Stieglitz was awarded a Fulbright Fellowship and assigned to Laos, leading to his career with the Foreign Service in which he held such posts as Cultural Attaché in Bangkok and in Brussels. He has also served as Washington correspondent for the *Bangkok Post*.

9- 6/93